Language and Communication Intervention in Preschool Children

Ellenmorris Tiegerman-Farber

School for Language and Communication Development
North Bellmore, New York
Adelphi University
Garden City, New York

Allyn and Bacon
Boston • London • Toronto • Sydney • Tokyo • Singapore

To Jeremy and Jonathan Tiegerman, my sons and teachers.

To my four new children, Andrew, Douglas, Leslie, and Dana Farber.

To my husband, Joseph Farber.

To the School for Language and Communication Development and my students.

God bless you

Dr. Ellenmorris Tiegerman-Farber

A Simon & Schuster Company
Needham Heights, MA 02194

Series Editor: Kris Farnsworth
Editorial Assistant: Christine M. Shaw
Production Administrator: Joe Sweeney
Editorial-Production Service: Walsh Associates
Cover Administrator: Suzanne Harbison
Composition Buyer: Linda Cox
Manufacturing Buyer: Louise Richardson

Library of Congress Cataloging-in-Publication Data

Tiegerman, Ellenmorris
Language and communication intervention in preschool children / Ellenmorris Tiegerman.
p. cm.
Includes bibliographical references and index.
ISBN 0-02-420821-3
1. Language disorders in children—Treatment. 2. Communicative disorders in children—Treatment. I. Title.
RJ496.L35T54 1994
618.92'85506—dc20 94-6772
CIP

Printed in the United States of America
10 9 8 7 6 5 4 3 2 1 00 99 98 97 96 95

CONTENTS

PREFACE

After many years of university teaching and clinical practice, it has become obvious to me that children with language disorders are often misunderstood and misdiagnosed. For example, in New York State, the label Speech Impaired (which should have been Language Communication Disordered) was removed from the list of handicapping conditions for the preschool child. The fact that a state as large and "progressive" as New York does not recognize the label Language Communication Disordered is a frightening reality that affects thousands of children. Speech Language Pathologists have an important mission as advocates and teachers for this population.

I wrote this textbook with children with language communication disorders in mind. It emphasizes an intervention approach that is centered around school and family, rather than the clinical environment, and highlights such issues as the nature and needs of the child with language disorders; the role of the family and parent training in the child's education; the function of the classroom as a language laboratory; multicultural issues in education and assessment; and educational laws and procedures.

The first portion of the book (chapters 1–3) is dedicated to a description of the child with a language communication disorder, the role of the child's family, and the educational laws and procedures surrounding the child. The second portion of the book (chapters 4–7) focuses on the practical applications of intervention in the preschool setting, including identification and assessment of language communication disorders, a model of a clinical intervention program, and information regarding using the classroom as a laboratory and training the parent as a facilitator. Finally, the last chapter of the book (chapter 8) provides an anatomy of a successful school program, the School for Language and Communication Development (SLCD) in North Bellmore, New York.

"A Few Words from Toya Davis" is an important feature that you will find in every chapter. As a parent of a child with a language communication disorder, Mrs. Davis offers the reader a personalized view of experiences with the educational system and its changing demands. The case study of Mrs. Davis' son, Jonathan, is presented so that the student may focus more clearly on an individual child and his programmatic needs, since ultimately, education must be evaluated based upon its success with an individual child.

Speech language pathology is an exciting profession, offering a broad range of clinical opportunities. The challenge for our profession is to recognize its potential contribution to the field of education and to meet that challenge. My intent in writing this textbook was to reflect an educational vision for the future. I truly hope that the ideas, viewpoints, and clinical descriptions in it encourage students and teachers to discuss provocative issues.

ACKNOWLEDGMENTS

In acknowledging those who have helped in any endeavor in life, we acknowledge those who have given. At the outset, I would like to thank Ann Castel Davis, Administrative Editor, who supported this texbook project from its inception. I am grateful to Ann for her insights, her commitment, and her belief in me.

I would like to express my deepest appreciation to New York State Senator Dean G. Skelos, 9th District, for his staunch support of preschool children with language disorders. Senator Skelos led the battle for legislation in New York State for many years. His unswerving support of children with handicaps and their families clearly goes beyond the usual and the typical within the political process. Thousands of children and families have benefited from his work and belief in the early intervention process. As the Executive Director of the School for Language and Communication Development (SLCD), I will always be devoted to the Senator for his extraordinary support.

I would also like to thank Nassau County's Executive, Thomas S. Gulotta, who has worked diligently over the years to support SLCD on a daily basis. I cannot count the number of times that I have called upon the County Executive to assist me in operating, managing, and developing the School for Language and Communication Development. Through all of my tears and requests, he has never lost his patience or his sense of humor. The entire network system of preschool programs owes its very existence to Thomas S. Gulotta. I am grateful for representing one of his lead agencies in Nassau County. He has taught me a great deal over the years and I will always be devoted to him.

To my reviewers—Robert Ackerman, East Stroudsburg University of Pennsylvania; Anthony DeFeo, University of Arizona; Pamela S. Dutcher, Andrews University; Ronald Gillam, University of Texas at Austin; Karyn Bobkoff Katz, The University of Akron; and Libby Kumin, Loyola College—thank you for your comments, suggestions, and criticisms.

To the parents of SLCD, I acknowledge "God's road"—and the pain and the joy of walking that road. All of my stories and experiences of inspiration relate specifically to parents whom I have met and families with whom I have worked over the years. To all of them I say thank you for all the things that you have given, allowing me to share my life, my work, and your children. Thanks also to Lauren Rosen, who provided illustrations for the opening page of each chapter, and for the cover.

To the teachers and professionals at SLCD, you are the spirit and future of education. Your experiences at SLCD will truly be a cornerstone in your lives. Always challenge the system and never settle for anything less than excellence.

To SLCD's Board of Directors, often silent but always present, I thank you for your generous time, support, and commitment to a dream that became a reality. I express my deepest appreciation to Joseph Gnesin, Paul Rosen, Mark Weinstein, Toya Davis, Jimmy Sunshine, Robert DeMattia, Richard Goldstein, and Barry Neustein. Without your ongoing support, there would be no SLCD.

To Dr. Christine Radziewicz, Madeline Mando, Rosemarie King, Donna Aruta-Carella, Andrea Rieger, Toya Davis, and Dr. Stephen Cavallo, thank you for sharing my dream of SLCD. It has been wonderful working, fighting, and creating with you.

To Florence Lieber, my secretary, thank you for all your hard work and commitment.

To my parents, Morris and Rita Jacobs, I acknowledge that everything I have done represents a gift from you.

To my six children, Jeremy, Jonathan, Andrew, Douglas, Leslie, and Dana, I express my appreciation for your love, your patience, and your devotion to me as a mother. In being with the six of you, and loving you as I do, I express and fulfill the greatest part of myself.

Finally, to my husband Joseph Farber, who proposed to me in front of 200 families, teachers, and friends, I express my love, my devotion, and my commitment to life's challenges ahead.

CHAPTER

1

CHARACTERISTICS OF THE PRESCHOOL LANGUAGE-DISORDERED CHILD

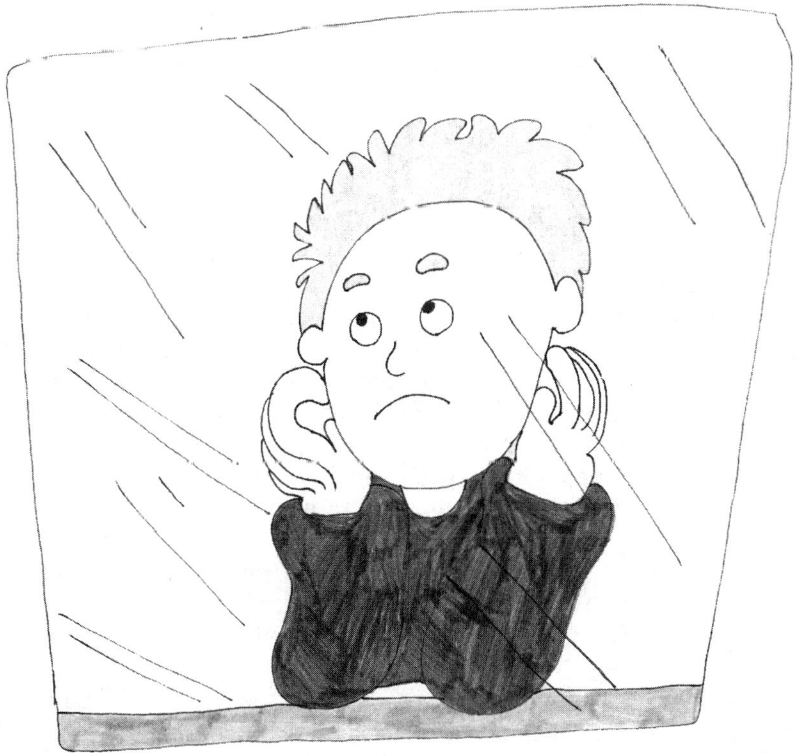

The area of child language development has progressed through a number of theoretical revolutions. Just as the underlying theoretical explanations of child language acquisition have changed, so, too, have intervention strategies. With child language theories as a primary framework, this chapter will discuss the learning characteristics and the unique learning needs of the language-disordered child. Each section will provide a short description of the developmental pattern in the normal language learner along with a discussion of intervention strategies.

In discussing the needs of any developmentally different population, it is important to understand the normal developmental model. Finally, it is the theoretical position of this author that children with developmental disabilities share a common problem—a pervasive language disorder—whatever the disabling conditions or educational labels. Specific learning characteristics of the language-disordered child may vary across populations, but the core components are shared. To the extent that the language needs are the same, the developmentally disordered child can be educated with other language-disordered children who present similar language needs. Although most educational-clinical programs are oriented toward a specific disabilities approach, the focus of this textbook is clearly in the opposite direction—a noncategorical-nonetiological approach to understanding developmentally disabled children. This certainly involves a change in "thinking and doing" at all operational levels—academic courses, clinical practice, and educational programming, to mention just a few. As with any revolution, someone needs to cross the line.

Etiological-Nonetiological Approaches

The professions dealing with speech/language pathology and the area of child language disorders have grown over the past three decades. The clinical techniques utilized in schools, hospitals, and speech and hearing centers have also changed dramatically as our perspective on the definition of *language* has expanded. There are two major approaches to the investigation and research of language and communication disorders in children: the etiological-categorical and the developmental-noncategorical.

The approach with which we are most familiar, particularly in the schools, involves classifying children with developmental disorders into specific categories. This approach is often likened to a medical model that emphasizes the relationship between distinct symptoms, a disease, and a specific medication or cure. In the medical model, it becomes very important to differentially diagnose the underlying physiological characteristics so that the medical practitioner can make an appropriate diagnosis; obviously, if the wrong medication is prescribed the patient will not get better.

An etiological-categorical approach has also been used in education. The original language of Public Law 94-142 lists specific disabling conditions, such as mental retardation, speech impairment, autism, and deafness. The etiological-categorical approach presents a rather convenient but simplistic means for identifying, classifying, and providing services for children with such disabilities. Each category functions as a label that allows children with the same deficit or difficulty to be educated together. The basic assumption of the etiological-categorical approach is that there are greater differences across classification categories than within the categories themselves; labels represent separate and distinct categories.

The use of labels has provided education with a streamlined mechanism to establish specific classes for children with different labels, e.g., classes for the autistic, classes for the mentally retarded, and classes for the deaf. In fact, many parents have advocated aggressively for children's services based upon specific labels. In many states, services provided to autistic children are different from the services provided for mentally retarded children. Many special educators feel that the labels ensure homogeneity in classroom programming and curriculum development. When all the children in a specific class have the same educational label, it becomes much easier to ensure that each child's individual needs will be met. Basically, this approach highlights the fact that special education programming has often been designed with the notion of etiology in mind; curricula, tests, and therapy materials are meant for the mentally retarded child, for example. A critical question, however, is whether children with different clinical labels are significantly different from one another. Do the labels provide an important learning dimension to the education of children with different disabling conditions?

As the definition of *language* has changed, the use and efficacy of the etiological-categorical approach has been questioned. Children with developmental disabilities often cannot be pigeonholed into specific categories. The underlying basic assumption, which is perfectly appropriate for a medical model, has not been shown to be appropriate in education. The developmental-noncategorical approach suggests that there are more differences within a developmental category than across developmental categories; the categories are *not* distinct. This approach proposes that we do not have in education highly distinct and separate groupings of children. Children classified as mentally retarded may also be hearing impaired. Children with cerebral palsy may be mentally retarded and hearing impaired. And, even though children may share characteristics, the causes of their underlying impairments may be different. Perhaps the placement of children by label or educational category is no longer meaningful; homogeneity may not serve an appropriate function if it is determined by etiology.

When all the children in a specific class have the same educational label, it may *not* be possible to ensure that each child's individual needs will be met, since there may be discrepancies in levels of functioning. Children with developmental disabilities share a more basic developmental problem: They all have a language disorder. It may be more efficacious and efficient in educational programming to consider the descriptive characteristics of the child's lan-

Figure 1–1
The Direct Causal Model Compared to the Shared Base Model

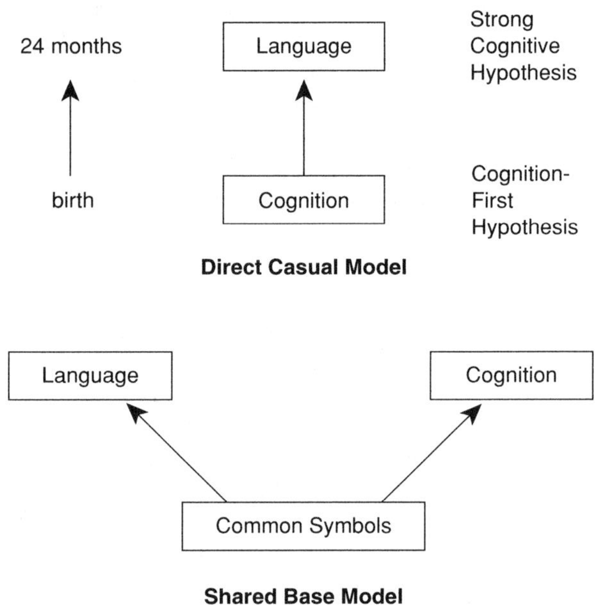

guage learning needs rather than his or her label. The notion here is that two children who have the same label can be at two different levels of functioning; one child may be nonverbal, and the other highly verbal. Should these two mentally retarded children be placed in the same class? Do they have the same educational needs?

If classroom assignment and educational programming represent the most important decision in this process, the child's language learning level may be a primary factor or characteristic to consider. Why not classify children by the type of language disorder? Why not group children and establish classrooms based on language level or language learning needs? There is much to be said for the developmental-noncategorical approach to education; it focuses on language characteristics and provides a common thread for classroom-based instruction. It also provides for specific programming and remediation that is transdisciplinary in nature and can be generalized from special education teacher to speech/language pathologist to occupational therapist.

Language represents a symbolic representational system that provides the underpinning for all areas of academic instruction. It is probably the most important tool that a child acquires. The present text suggests that children with developmental disabilities all share a common problem—a language disorder. In understanding the area of language disorders, education itself is empowered to look at children through a common telescope and see to it that (1) all children are described, classified, and educated in terms of their language learning needs; (2) a language curriculum becomes the basis for educational instruction; and (3) all professionals access the same terminology, curriculum technology, and transdisciplinary approach. This text proposes that an understanding of language provides a powerful approach for future educational programming. Language represents the one system and tool that can allow for decision making for *all* children in the educational system—disabled and nondisabled alike.

Reconsidering Language and Cognition

Historically, the cognitive viewpoint has been Piagetian in approach. This means that as professionals—teachers, educators, and parents—we thought that cognition as a general developmental area was acquired first. It also means that cognition was primary and language was based on cognitive skills (see Figure 1–1). This is frequently referred to in the literature as the Direct Causal Model. As the definition of language changed over the past three decades, researchers began to find that normal children acquired language abilities at much younger ages. One of the most important theoretical and clinical investigations was performed by Bates, Benigni, Bretherton, Camaioni, and Volterra (1979)—they documented the development of referential language in children between *eight* and *ten* months of age. This created quite a flurry in the research literature, ultimately resulting in what has now been accepted as a shift in the relationship between language and cognition. Most researchers in the field of child language development today argue that not only does language occur much earlier than Piaget proposed, but that it is *not* dependent on cognitive abilities or structures (i.e., developmental homologies). This more recent model (the Shared Base Model) suggests that language and cognition develop from a common set of symbols interdependently.

Since the relationship between language and cognition has changed, we now look at the child development process very differently. Researchers understand that the most important developmental occurrence between birth and four years of age involves the acquisition of the language system. This has clinical import for the disabled child, early intervention, and curriculum programming. Language involves a complex system (see Figure 1–2) that includes a number of developmental components: pragmatics, semantics, and syntax. Language represents the child's most critical accomplishment during the early childhood years; *all* academic subjects, *all* educational instruction, *all* later acquisitions are based on the language learning system. A child cannot be tested without language. A child cannot read without language. A child cannot learn social studies, science, or health education without language.

Language involves a system of symbols that a child requires for communication and socialization. For a child without the ability to talk and communicate, the prognosis for independent functioning is poor. The research indicates that there is a formative or critical period for language learning (a biological time clock). If functional language is not acquired by the age of five, the probability

Figure 1–2
The Language Model

Components	Functional Elements
FORM	*Phonology* Rules that govern speech sounds and their combinations. *Morphology* Rules that govern the internal organization of words. *Syntax* Rules that govern the word order, sentence structure, and organization.
CONTENT	*Semantics* Rules that govern the meaning of words and their combinations.
USE	*Pragmatics* Rules relating to the use of language in social contexts.

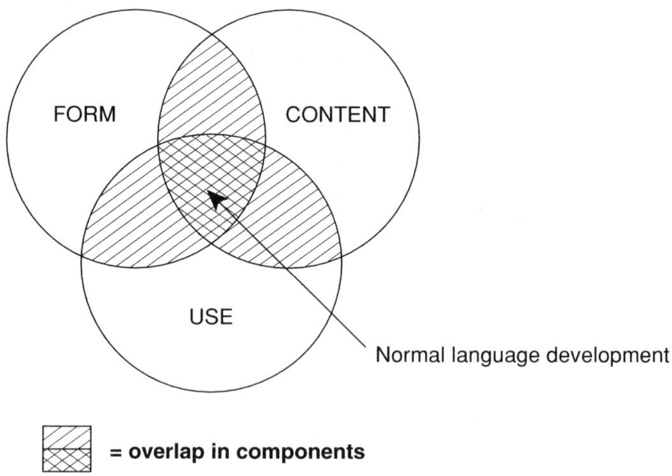

Source: L. Bloom & M. Lahey, *Language Development and Language Disorders*. New York: Wiley, 1978.

for normal language decreases dramatically for each six months of life. After age eight, there is almost no chance for the child to acquire a normal language system, that is, a symbolic representational system. It is not surprising, therefore, that the research literature emphasizes the significance of early identification and intervention for disabled children. The earlier the initiation of intervention services, the smaller the educational problems over time, and the less severe the child's difficulties will be. The later the initiation of intervention, the more serious the child's problems become and the more costly the resulting programming.

Language Components

An investigation of the research literature on child development issues highlights the fact that the definition of *language* has changed significantly in the past thirty years. In the 1960s it focused on the acquisition of syntactic structures; in the 1970s it expanded to include the acquisition of syntax (language structure) *and* semantics (language meaning). In the 1980s it expanded again to include a third component and to give us our present definition of language—syntax (language structure), semantics (language meaning), *and* pragmatics (language function) (see Figure 1–2). These three language components are acquired in a steplike or stagelike fashion in the first thirty-six months of life (see Figure 1–3). After thirty-six months the child goes about the business of not only integrating all of the language information that he or she has acquired, but also integrating that information with other developmental areas.

Language learning occurs along a developmental continuum. Perhaps the analogy of a tree would help to elucidate this language-learning process in children (see Figure 1–4). The tree diagram indicates that each language component—pragmatics (communication), semantics (meaning), and syntactics

Figure 1–3
Language Component Steps

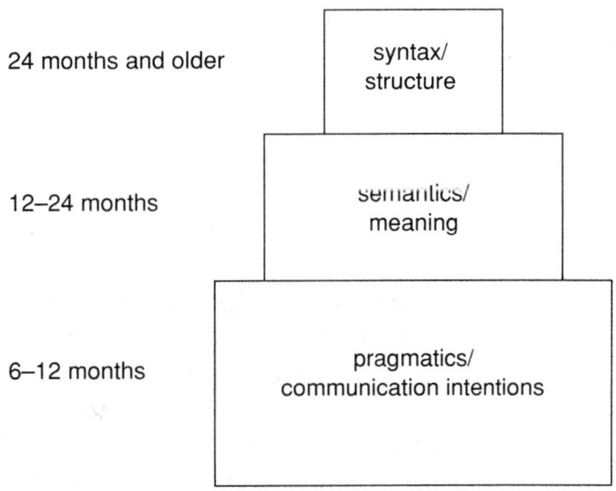

Figure 1–4
The Tree of Language Integration

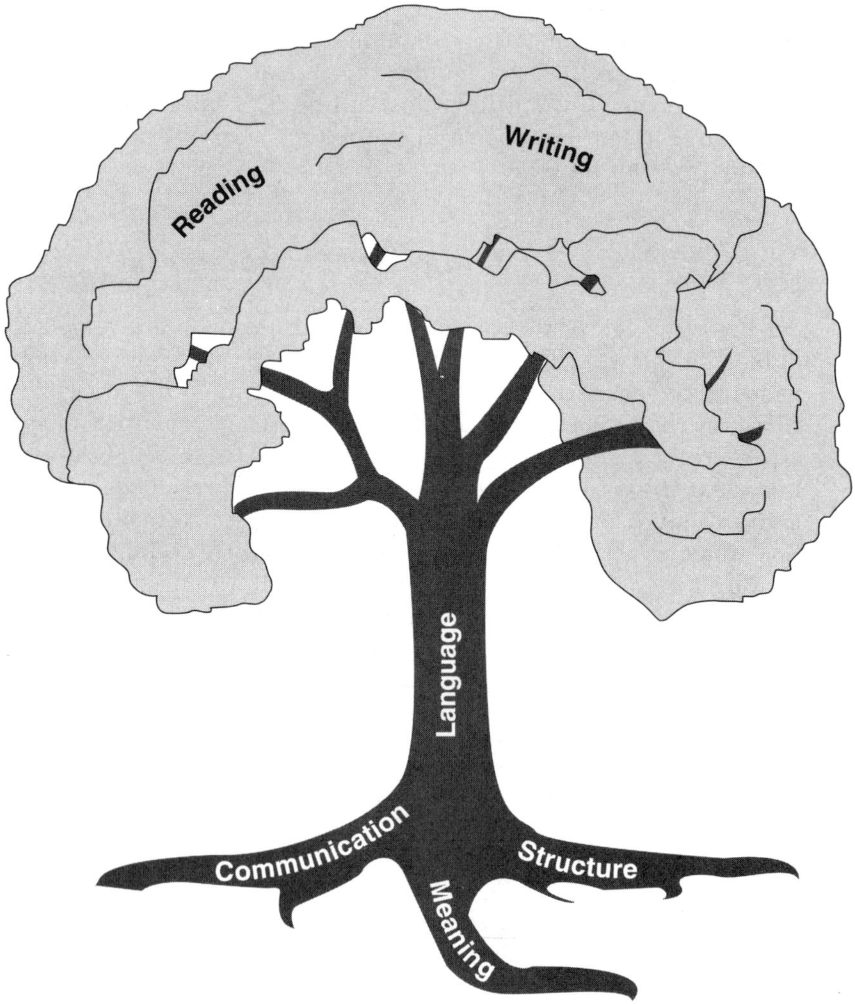

(structure)—represents a root embedded firmly and deeply in the earth. The embedding aspect reflects the fact that when the roots are not deeply embedded, the tree's growth is impaired; shallow roots result in a tree that leans or topples as it matures. The language components or roots during early development combine and interface to form a tree trunk. Again, if the roots of the tree are weak, there is risk that the entire tree will fall over and/or develop a range of growth problems—in this case, language problems. When a language disorder is present, there is a problem in one or more of the language roots. The language components feed the language system, just as the roots feed the tree. When the earlier developmental skills are impaired, later abilities are negatively affected; for example, early semantic developmental deficits may result in word-finding difficulties and reading problems later in school.

Most speech/language pathologists use the model in Figure 1–2 to explain the components of language that are acquired during the formative period of early development. Language involves the ability to use a conventional system consisting of arbitrary symbols in order to generate ideas for the purposes of communication. Language is a code, a representational system that a child uses to interact with and exchange information with others. To communicate, the child must develop a conceptual understanding of the communication process, a knowledge of the context, and understanding of speaker and of listener roles as well as a repertoire of interactional behaviors. The ability to modify the interactional process, share, and exchange information requires learning and integration of developmental skills (Prizant & Wetherby, 1990).

The definition of *language* includes the component areas that will be discussed in this chapter: pragmatics (language use), semantics (language content), syntax, morphology, and phonology (language structure). Normal language development involves the ability to integrate these component areas. Language integration or the integration of language skills is an important learning ability. The entire language system may be compared to an orchestra. Each part of the orchestra has its own distinct instruments and sound: the woodwinds, the brass, the strings, and the percussion instruments. Each section creates its own sound but in the context of a symphony the sections must play in harmony. It is this harmonious blending of the sounds of the instruments that produces the majesty of the symphony. The integration of language skills can be compared to the interactional process that occurs in an orchestra. When the language system is intact, skills are blended across the language component areas, and there is a learning harmony in the normal language learner.

In the language-disordered child, each section plays independently of the others, and sounds across the orchestra are not timed or tuned with regard to a symphonic composition. As a result, the music created is cacophonous, or disharmonious. Development within component areas appears to be independent rather than interdependent. Information and learning do not interface with developments in other areas. Acquisition in some children appears to be sectional rather than holistic and generalizable to other areas. At times development appears to be not only disharmonious but also erratic. It is essential to understand the normal language learner (the harmonious symphonic production) in order to understand the language-disordered child (the disharmonious symphonic production).

The American Speech-Language and Hearing Association's definition of language disorders is:

> A language disorder is the abnormal acquisition, comprehension, or expression of spoken or written language. The disorder may involve all, one, or some of the phonologic, morphologic, semantic, syntactic, or pragmatic components of the linguistic system. Individuals with language disorders frequently have problems in sentence processing or in abstracting information meaningfully for storage and retrieval from short- and long-term memory (ASHA, 1980, pp. 317–318).

ASHA's definition notes three important guidelines for considering language disorders: the components of language that might be impaired, the modalities that might be impaired, and the processes that might be impaired.

Bloom and Lahey (1978) described the following characteristics:

1. Children exhibit difficulties in learning linguistic form. They indicate difficulties in understanding and using phonological, morphological, and syntactic rules.
2. Children exhibit difficulties in conceptualization and formulation of ideas about objects, events, and relations.
3. Children exhibit difficulties in language use. They cannot regulate their language structures to meet the listener's needs. They cannot use language to convey a range of communicative functions, and they have difficulties in understanding and speaking in social contexts.

The following sections are presented to contrast and to highlight normal language aspects, disordered language aspects, and intervention strategies. Since this is not a textbook on normal language development, there are many processes that are not discussed. The purpose here is to provide the student, the teacher, and the special educator with comparative themes across these areas that will generate discussion on how these areas are related to one another. These sections are not meant to be definitive in their research or clinical dimensions; the contrast represents a process of inquiry and analysis.

A language disorder is the abnormal acquisition, comprehension, or production of spoken or written language (ASHA, 1980, pp. 317–318), resulting in pragmatic, semantic, and syntactic deficits.

Language Use

Normal Pragmatic Abilities

Children learn to communicate various intentions (i.e., request, comment, protest, negate) long before they develop linguistic abilities (specifically, the structures that relate to the conventional code: sound, word, and sentence). During the first twelve months of life, children communicate their intentions by using a combination of gaze, vocal, and gestural behaviors. During this period of prelinguistic behavior, the context plays an important role in helping the adult to interpret the child's meaning. Gaze + point + vocalization + gesture + context are all used by the parent to figure out what the child wants. The child develops the ability to express a range of communicative intentions by combining and recombining the behaviors in his or her repertoire. Although there are a limited number of behaviors in that repertoire, communicative understanding occurs because of the interactional contingencies for parent and child. Although initially the child is not aware of the impact of his or her behavior, the contingent and consistent responding of the parent is critical in teaching the child to communicate. In the process of becoming aware of being a communicator, the child replaces the idiosyncratic forms of communication with the more conventional structures of the language environment.

During this social learning period, children also have the ability to engage in proto-conversational exchanges with adults. Prototypical conversation does not involve the use of words; instead, it involves a complex sequence of looking or gaze interactions. Later the conversation with the eyes will include words and sentences. These behaviors and interactions are important to later language skills because they provide a framework. Discourse skills have their roots in these early gaze interactional conversations. This developmental pattern highlights the progression and the importance of communicative forms and functions. Normal infants are spontaneous, imitative, inquisitive, and interactive as learners. They actively contribute to the communication process and are perceived as a communicator and partner by their mothers. During the first stage, the children are communicative but not linguistic. By the end of the first year of life, they have acquired the foundation for later linguistic development—communicative interaction. The normal developmental pattern underscores the significance of communication to later language acquisition—communication comes first.

During the preschool years, children expand their communicative intentions by means of social interactions with peers and adults. As children interact and socialize, they practice the use of their pragmatic language functions. This is an example of how *learning to learn* provides preschoolers with the ability to be better communicators. Preschool children learn how to manage different social settings and different social communicators. They learn how to function as speakers as well as listeners. In becoming effective social communicators, preschool children learn to express their wants and needs across a range of contexts and people. They learn to take turns in conversation. They learn to provide relevant information. They learn to ask questions. The development of language use becomes progressively more complex. As children progress through their preschool years and become effective social communicators, they learn not only to express their own needs but also to attune themselves sensitively to the needs of others.

The Language-Disordered Child

The preschool child with pragmatic deficits presents the following communicative/interactional problems: (1) does not develop a range of communicative functions; (2) does not develop gaze interaction skills; (3) does not develop prototypical behaviors such as protodeclaratives or protoimperatives; (4) does not develop attention and joint action schemes; (5) does not develop an awareness of agent, action, or object contingencies; (6) does not develop turn-taking or reciprocal action skills; and (7) does not develop gestures or imitation behaviors. Lack of eye contact, avoidance of social contexts and physical contacts, noncommunicative gestures and facial expressions, and mutism are some of the characteristics that are often described.

The prelinguistic behaviors such as pointing, showing, or turn-taking are typically not present. As a result, the development of communicative behavior in language-disordered children is different from the normal developmental sequence. Most do not develop a range of communicative functions; as a result their communicative and social interactions are limited. Social context facilitates learning in normal children; language-disordered children, however, often avoid social interactions. They remove themselves from the very contexts that they need to teach themselves about communication. Given their severe communication deficits, improving their social functioning should be of primary importance to their families and educators.

Normal communicative development does not occur consecutively from one function to another; some functions emerge concurrently (Wetherby, 1986). Linguistic structures develop from communicative functions; children talk about the here and now, and they talk about their experiences in the interactional context. It is the social context that provides the basis for the development of conversational forms. In contrast to the synchronous development of communicative functions by normal children, it appears that language-disordered children may acquire the functions of language one at a time. This suggests that the communicative pattern developed is qualitatively as well as quantitatively different from the normal prelinguistic sequence. Disordered children may acquire communicative functions in a different developmental sequence and, as a result, their linguistic abilities will be different. Prizant and Wetherby (1987) describe the following communicative characteristics: (1) communicative intent in gestural and vocal areas develops asynchronously; (2) communicative profile is different from that in other children; (3) the sequence of communicative development is different; (4) the repertoire of communicative functions is limited; (5) certain aberrant behaviors can be intentional, interactive, and communicative; and (6) there is limited development of behaviors that result in a social consequence.

The description of the language-disordered child as noncommunicative and noninteractive is not accurate. Such a child, even one with a limited range of communicative behaviors, responds differently to different interactional partners. So it is not the case that he does not interact, but rather that his range of communicative options is limited. Another factor that interferes with the language-disordered child's communicative effectiveness involves her idiosyncratic behaviors. Whereas the normal language learner develops conventional behaviors to communicate needs, the language-disordered child may utilize behaviors that are not standard linguistic forms. The result is that the social communicators in the child's environment may misinterpret and misunderstand her intentions and her meaning. Bernard-Opitz (1982) suggests that the communication context is important to the language-disordered child and the adults in her environment. The context provides a mechanism for adults to disambiguate the child's meaning. Adults can figure out what the child is attempting to communicate by combining a number of fragments: vocalization + action + context (i.e., just as one would have to do with a very young normal language learner).

Communication Intervention Strategies

The context is important for therapeutic intervention. Program goals should be designed to expand the language-disordered child's communicative intentions by using natural and functional aspects of the environment. It is also suggested that the child's communicative abilities can only be determined by analyzing behaviors in an interactional situation with social partners. This analysis would highlight (1) the communicative acts used by adult and child; (2) the relationship between spontaneous and echolalic utterances; (3) the number of conversational topics and resulting turns on each topic; and (4) the child's communicative differences as a function of different partners and contexts. Communication goals should be a primary component of programming for the language-disordered child. In order to develop such goals, however, the language disorder must be assessed in various communication contexts.

Beisler and Tsai (1983) studied the development of communicative functions in five language-disordered children. The authors note that pragmatic communicative functions should be facilitated rather than the use of specific linguistic forms or structures. One problem related to the child's learning style is that linguistic forms may be acquired as routinized chunks. Historically, clinical and educational programs have focused on teaching specific linguistic structures or forms. The result has been the rigid reproduction of these "frozen" strings or phrases without a semantic-syntactic understanding of the utterances. Educators need to observe more closely how the normal child develops communication, social, and language skills.

Normal children learn about communication by experiencing a communicative process of joint action and joint attention. The language-disordered child needs to experience the same communicative process and to participate in the same kind of facilitative social context. Programs should incorporate a pragmatic approach to teaching the function of language-communication. Clearly, the communication deficit is quite evident from the child's inability to have a conversation and his inability to engage in reciprocal interaction. The authors recommend that intervention should be communication-based: (1) teach the child to take turns during dyadic interaction; (2) activities should be child-directed and child-centered; (3) adult input should be semantically related and regulated to the child's level of comprehension; (4) communicative interaction should be the first and primary goal—with or without verbal language.

Communicative intentions can be stimulated and established by natural obstacles within the context. Educators should introduce activities that will engage the child in actions and object manipulation. They should choose objects based on the child's interests and preferences. The emphasis in learning should be through shared transactional experiences and *talking* about what is happening in the immediate situation. Situational routines provide the child with a learned format that can then be manipulated by means of an obstacle that breaks the routine. The clinician could provide a model by producing what the child might say in the situation. In addition, the child's name should be used instead of personal pronouns, which can be confusing. Wetherby (1986) suggests that educational techniques must take into consideration the language-disordered child's communication learning style. Training procedures that focus on imitating linguistic strings that are reinforced with primary reinforcers such as food may be counterproductive to learning. The language-disordered child should be taught language in a natural communicative context. Communicative situations can be devised around the child's interests and object preferences, using naturally occurring events such as bathing, dressing, eating, and playing.

Prizant and Wetherby (1987) propose that intentionality must combine with conventionality to develop communication. A close analysis of communicative intent might highlight the social and communicative dysfunctions in the language-disordered child; she may not use conventional forms such as pointing or showing to express communicative intentions. Idiosyncratic behaviors such as echolalia and self-stimulation (highly repetitive and perseverative performances) may be used to signal various communicative functions. One assumption is that because the child does not use conventional forms of communication, she cannot communicate. This position may be as inappropriate as the one that assumes that the language-disordered child's use of conventional forms reflects an intention to communicate. The meaning of the child's interaction can only be determined by analyzing his or her behavior in the social context. Analyzing unconventional communicative forms and functions requires multiple observations across different contexts. The authors note that the ultimate challenge is to determine if the unconventional forms actually express communicative intentions.

A pragmatic approach focuses on communication learning first in language. It highlights the significance of the social environment in facilitating interaction between the child and the adult and between peers. The naturally occurring events that constitute classroom and home experiences provide a rich source of learning. The roles and rules of communication can best be learned in a social context in which the child participates and experiences the consequences of his or her behavior. Learning to communicate can only occur in a social environment. For the language-disordered child, the social environment must be structured and organized to facilitate the communicative process.

JONATHAN

Jonathan has been enrolled at the School for Language and Communication Development for the past year; he is presently three years, six months old. Jonathan can be described by the following characteristics. He presents with a severe language and communication disorder affecting pragmatic, semantic, and syntactic components of language. His eye gaze interactions appear limited, along with his turn-taking skills and attending behaviors. He demonstrates limited abilities in following directions, coding communicative interactions, and responding to other communicators. Jonathan's language production consists primarily of echolalic verbalizations.

In the classroom setting, Jonathan's overall pragmatic skills are below age-level expectancies. He requires maximal prompting to maintain eye contact with peers and adults during structured and unstructured activities. Jonathan is highly distractible, and he often loses focus. As activities become more complex, he demonstrates deficits in his ability to attend to structured and unstructured activities. When he becomes distractible, he often self-stimulates by flapping his hands, walking away from the activity, and/or by singing to himself. Often he focuses on internal stimuli and appears to gaze fixedly at a moving object. He requires verbal and physical prompting to complete even simple activities. He appears to have less difficulty attending to object-related activities that have a high degree of repetition, such as puzzles and blocks.

Jonathan demonstrates difficulty with verbal and nonverbal turn-taking skills, since he is highly echolalic. There is a marked difference between his echolalic utterances (MLU 7-10.0 and spontaneous productions < 1.0). His delayed echolalic productions consist of commercials, jingles, and utterances that he has heard at home. He utilizes a monotonic intonational pattern except when he gets frustrated; then he begins to screech. Jonathan requires verbal prompts and models to code the pragmatic functions of regulating, commenting, and protesting. He has not begun to utilize the pragmatic functions of describing, commenting, and interpreting.

Jonathan does not initiate verbal or nonverbal interactions with peers or adults. He demonstrates difficulty maintaining teacher- or peer-initiated exchanges. Jonathan does not exhibit conversational abilities or narrative skills at this time. He cannot elaborate or provide descriptive information. His responses are consistently rote and predictable. Since he has difficulty expressing a range of communicative functions, his communication interactions and play behaviors tend to be routinized and stereotypic. Jonathan tends to stand on the periphery of a peer group and often retreats when approached by another child. He becomes easily overstimulated in group situations and often requires transitional objects as he moves from therapy session to therapy session. He is often communicatively unrelated to the ongoing context.

Pragmatic Goals

1. To establish appropriate eye gaze behaviors.
2. To increase the use of pragmatic functions presently in the child's repertoire.
3. To increase communicative interaction by acquiring new pragmatic functions.
4. To demonstrate turn-taking skills in conversational exchange and play interactions.
5. To increase object-related interactions in play sequences.
6. To increase nonverbal initiations and interactions in naturally occurring activities.

LANGUAGE CONTENT

Normal Semantic Abilities

The second year of life is distinguished by the development of wordlike utterances that are embedded in jargonlike productions. These utterances are quite distinctive as long strings that carry sentential intent; that is, they carry the force of a sentencelike structure. The wordlike structures more closely approximate the conventional linguistic forms of the language; the forms used by the child to communicate intentions expand to include wordlike structures along with gestures. The child learns that the more closely he approximates the linguistic structures, the more effectively he functions as a communicator. Quickly, the child becomes aware that the *word* is more efficient than a series of vocalizations, gestures, and points.

The child's earliest intentions relate to his own individual and specific needs as the linguistic is mapped onto the nonlinguistic and the verbal mapped onto the nonverbal. The word replaces the gesture and the vocalization in the expression of communicative intentions (requesting, commenting, showing, and rejecting) and becomes linguistic structures, conventional forms. As the child interacts with his environment there are cognitive and semantic developments as well. His manipulative and interactive experiences give rise to three conceptual notions that establish the foundation for semantic relationships: agents (people), actions (doing), and objects (manipulandum). These broad conceptual ideas represent the content of child language.

The content of a child's language expresses his understanding of the relationships among agents, actions, and objects. Her experiences in the environment—the nonlinguistic context—teach her about the relationships between people and objects, actions and objects, and people and actions. At first, she talks about her own world and her own needs. At this stage, her language is concrete in its meaning; it is contextually specific and contextually bound to the immediate environment. She can only talk about the *here and now;* she has not developed to a level of decontextualization. The area of semantics is defined as meaning encoded in language. Children at this stage begin to learn the relationship between meaning and structure. They learn that meaning can be expressed by certain linguistic forms. The normal child learns that words, phrases, sentences, and stories have meaning. The object of this stage is learning to mean.

As children develop linguistic forms, they express the functions of language in more conventional ways. Learning to mean takes many years and begins during infancy when the baby uses gaze and vocal behavior to interact and communicate with parents. By the end of the first twelve months, children add wordlike utterances to their gestural repertoire. When they finally produce word combinations, they use the formal conventional structures of a language. They learn that meaning changes over time. As they add new experiences, their insights change and word meaning expands. There is, therefore, a critical relationship between the development of meaning and what a child means by what he says—and a child's experiences in the world. As meaning becomes more sophisticated, it is also extended as it is analyzed and interpreted within the framework of a sentence or a photograph or a story. Children are often asked "What is the main idea?" or "What is the moral to the story?" In the process of extracting the meaning from a story, the child must be able to step away from the material and understand that meaning transcends the structure of language.

There are several different theories of semantic development. These theories are neither exhaustive nor exclusive; they are presented to highlight the diversity of ideas related to semantic development in children. All of these theories may interact and play a role in the child's development of meaning. It is interesting to consider and to observe how different children appear to have preferences in their approaches to learning about their environment. Perhaps these theories represent learning styles or preferences in children as they acquire content knowledge about their world. All of the theories suggest that as children continue to experience reality, their ideas and concepts about objects and events change.

Semantic Feature Hypothesis

Clark (1973) proposed the Semantic Feature Hypothesis. An object in the environment consists of a number of features and characteristics that the child perceives. The child must determine which features and characteristics are relevant in determining the boundaries of category meaning given a specific referent. Children appear to identify the most salient characteristics, which in turn define what the word means. Since children have a very limited range of experiences, their definition for a word is much narrower or more restricted than the adult's meaning for that same word. A thirty-month-old may define a "doggie" as a four-legged creature. In the process of identifying all four-legged creatures as "doggie," he learns that there are other characteristics such as "meow," establishing a cat category, and "oink, oink," establishing a pig category. The overgeneralization in meaning represents a very early strategy that provides him with a great deal of adult feedback. The important point, however, is that the child's meaning is quite different from the adult's meaning.

Functional Core Hypothesis

Nelson (1974) suggested another theory that described the development of child meaning. Here, the child bases her word concept on her active relationship with an object rather than on perceptual characteristics. The child's definition is directly a function of what she does with the object. This suggests that early explorations through direct manipulation provide the foundation for meaning development; the conceptual aspects of a child's experience appear to be related to early semantic language development.

Prototype Hypothesis

Bowerman (1978) suggested that the child develops a prototype that provides a mechanism for comparison. The prototype incorporates a child's concept for "a chair." All other objects that share these characteristics or features are then compared to this mental representation. The closer the exemplar is to the prototype concept, the greater the likelihood that the child will refer to it by that lexical entry or label.

These three theories of semantic development all suggest possibilities in terms of how a child's meaning changes conceptually over time and approaches the adult's meaning. It also appears that there are many consistencies cross-culturally and cross-linguistically, indicating that children develop the same semantic relationships all over the world. This seems to suggest that, despite obvious linguistic differences, children learn to express the same ideas about agents, actions, and objects wherever they live. Despite the environmental differences across cultures, it is quite remarkable that relationships—semantic relationships—are highly similar.

Vocabulary Development

During the preschool years, children acquire a vocabulary, or lexicon. A child's vocabulary reflects his experiences in his environment and his knowledge about the world. His first words are nouns and verbs—labels for objects and actions that are most salient to him. The most interesting change in lexical development occurs with the acquisition of grammatical morphemes, which will be discussed in the next section. Morphological inflections begin to appear at the end of the second year of life with the occurrence of word combinations.

Children initially express an idea or proposition by using single words embedded in social and gestural structures. As the lexicon increases, they use multiword constructions to express a single proposition. During the third year of life, they join clauses and phrases to form longer units of meaning into different sentence types. They combine adult linguistic information with personal environmental interactions. Experiences with objects, people, actions, and events provide a source of learning about words and meanings. As children's experiences vary and expand, their knowledge of objects, people, actions, and events changes. As this nonlinguistic knowledge changes, so do word meanings.

A word is a conceptual category; it transcends any single experience. A word is a symbol because it represents a number of characteristics and descriptions. Concepts are formed as experiences change the child's perceptions of an object, an action, or an event. As new knowledge is integrated into the lexical system, an internal representation of a word is generated. As the child's knowledge of the social environment (nonlinguistic context) broadens, so also does her word (linguistic) meaning expand. When experiential or world knowledge is expressed through language, it becomes semantic rather than cognitive knowledge. The preschool language learner constructs both linguistic and nonlinguistic categories. Linguistic categories include concepts about words (vocabulary) and relationships between words (syntactic constructions that convey meaning). Experience changes meaning and these changes in language ultimately alter the experiential learning process.

Processing Styles

As meaning changes, old knowledge provides a framework for processing new information. Normal language learners utilize two styles of information processing—gestalt and analytic. The gestalt style allows the child to learn an entire sentence or paragraph as a chunk or a unit without the necessity of breaking down the linguistic production into component elements. This allows the child to combine a linguistic structure or utterance as a chunk with an event. With the analytic style, new information can be compared to old information for the purpose of concept development, specifically semantic concepts. The analytic processing style allows the child to break the message down into meaning units based on past experiences.

Hubbell (1981) suggested that semantic memory involves the ability to conceptualize beyond any single or specific context. Here the child abstracts relevant information across situations to organize concepts for long-term memory. Semantic knowledge refers to the meaning encoded in language. This semantic ability would allow the child to symbolically represent and reconstruct an event. Hubbell noted that in order "to learn language a child must be able to reconstruct sentences, not merely recite them" (p. 29). The analytic style allows for generation with an understanding of meaning and internal structure of utterances. In normal development, the two styles operate together and interface to facilitate the language learning process.

Extending Meaning

The most advanced structures for the expression of meaning involve the extension beyond the sentence, that is, narration and conversation. Kintsch (1974) describes how common events become organized into scripts by children. As they begin to understand the organization of events and learn to conceptualize a sequence within the event, they start to describe this sequence in script form. Duchan (1986) suggests that the narrative experience is facilitated through conversational exchange. In learning to interact with an adult in a conversational format, a child describes a personal experience sequentially with details and outcomes. During this exchange, the child learns to function both as a speaker and as a listener. He is required to explain, remain relevant to the topic, adjust his behavior to his listener, and respond to questions. There are specific rules that govern conversational exchange and narrative structures, and each has its own semantic and developmental format and function.

Discourse Skills

Learning to have a conversation represents an important and complex social process. The ability to have a conversation involves a set of interactional skills that become much more sophisticated as the child's language becomes more complex. Preschool children must learn to share information dyadically on a specific topic. This means that the child must learn to listen to a peer, provide new information, stay on topic, and take her turn appropriately. There are specific roles and rules related to conversational exchange. The roles involve learning how to be an effective speaker and listener. This also means that in functioning in each of these roles there is a time to change from speaker to listener and from listener to speaker. Children have to learn when to allow someone else to speak. They must also learn not to interrupt another speaker. A conversation is very much like a dance; it involves two partners and a set of patterned steps. If the conversation is going to be meaningful, the two partners must remain in synchrony. In a conversation children must learn to listen to their partner and provide information that is related and relevant, but not repetitious. Obviously, if one partner speaks out of turn, "someone's toes will be stepped on," and the dance will stop.

Learning to have a conversation is an important semantic and developmental skill. During the preschool years, children learn to fine-tune this skill so that the number of exchanges or turns on a topic increase as the child's language becomes more complex. The ability to describe in detail present and past events becomes more specific. Having a conversation also allows the preschool child the opportunity to ask questions and explore the world by means of verbal language. Preschool children learn that there are many things they cannot experience, but they can ask questions about an event in a book, on television, or in a song. This provides a means of acquiring additional information about agents, actions, and objects in the world around them. Having a conversation allows them to share feelings and thoughts, and provides an important language-learning lesson—extending and expanding content knowledge by using the language system.

Narrative Skills

The narrative process is probably facilitated through natural conversational exchange. During conversational interaction, the preschooler describes events and experiences as well as sequences and outcomes. This provides the beginnings of a simple narrative sequence. A narration is simply a description of the child's personal experiences and perceptions of the world; it reflects her basic knowledge and understanding of linguistic and nonlinguistic relationships. A narration is a story sequence that allows the preschool child to detail some personal occurrence that was meaningful during the daily routine. The child's daily experiences are generally organized around events that are action-based. Over time these common events become organized scripts because they are familiar and they occur over and over again. This process of experiential reoccurrence allows the child to elaborate the organized script into anticipated outcomes and recognizable sequences—language chunks of information.

As preschool children begin to understand that events can be organized into a script, the story narrative becomes conceptualized into linguistically coded elements. Yoshinaga-Itano and Downey (1986) report that children develop narrative or story scripts so that they learn to embed one schematic representation within another. A story narrative is a monologue, not a conversation. In a conversation there are a number of turns between speaker and listener as information is exchanged on a specific topic. In a narration, the topic is the story and the story is presented by the speaker for the purpose of detailing a specific event. The relationship, therefore, between the speaker and the listener is quite different. In a narration, it is the speaker's role to provide all the information; the listener's role involves paying attention to the details of the story without interrupting the storyteller. It is often interesting to note that children must learn the difference between conversation and narration. Preschool children must learn to adjust their language behaviors and messages not only to individual communication partners, topics, and contexts, but also to the purpose of the interaction—conversation or narration. Narration, like conversation, reflects the child's knowledge base and understanding of her world through her descriptive detail and analysis.

The language system provides a mechanism for the child to learn language by using language. The more he uses his language system the better he becomes at it—learning to learn. In this case, he becomes more effective at learning to mean; the process of meaning becomes internalized and conceptualized in the child—meaning to mean. The child realizes there is a process to knowledge acquisition. He can engage in the process as an exercise for learning or for the sheer enjoyment of *word play.*

The Language-Disordered Child

The child with a language disorder may not comprehend or produce meaning by means of the normal developmental pattern; as a result he or she may be a language chunker and utilize a gestalt style of language learning. The gestalt style results in the child's learning an entire sentence or paragraph as a unit without the benefit of analytic processing. This processing style helps to explain the occurrence of echolalia. In fact, echolalia itself represents a developmental advancement in a child who has just moved out of a long phase of mutism. He or she associates a sentence or phrase with a specific event; there is a rigid association between the linguistic and the nonlinguistic. The language-disordered child's semantic abilities can be assessed through an analysis of his or her echolalic behavior and how it changes progressively over time. The child's ability to change specific features in the imitative response is indicative of developing comprehension. As a result, it is important to discuss echolalia in order to understand its function in the language behavior of the language-disordered child.

Historically, *echolalia* has been defined as the meaningless repetition of a word or word group just spoken by another person (Fay, 1967). In examining the difference between the imitative pattern in normal and in language-disordered children, one finds that in the language-disordered child (1) the imitative utterances are longer, (2) the imitative utterances represent most of the child's repertoire, and (3) the imitative verbal behavior remains as a primary pattern for a longer period of time. For many years, behaviorists considered echolalia as interfering behavior that had to be extinguished; behavioral techniques were utilized to decrease the frequency of echolalic behaviors from the language-disordered child's repertoire. Recent developments in the area of child language research have described the language-disordered child's severe comprehension deficits. In the face of not understanding what has been said and not knowing how to respond, the language-disordered child does the best he can—he imitates.

Prizant and Duchan (1981) investigated how immediate echolalia functioned for children in interactions with familiar adults. *Immediate echolalia* is defined as an echolalic response that occurs subsequent to a speaker's utterance. The imitation must have structural similarities to the speaker's production. The data from their investigation indicated seven distinct categories of echolalia. For all of the subjects in the study, echolalic responses were produced more frequently with evidence of comprehension than without. Comprehension was based on the child's related and intentional actions immediately prior to, during, or after the production of the echolalic utterance. The meaning of the echolalic utterance was determined in terms of how it functioned for the child. Echolalia represents a transitional phase in the development of the child with a language disorder. Linguistic knowledge and comprehension can be measured by the child's ability to *change* syntactic structures and suprasegmental features. The authors suggest that echolalia must be studied as an integral part of the child's developing linguistic and cognitive abilities.

Prizant and Rydell (1984) investigated the functions of delayed echolalia in language-disordered children. *Delayed echolalia* refers to utterances repeated at a much later period of time. "Echolalic behaviors, both immediate and delayed, are best described as a continuum of behaviors in regard to exactness of repetition, degree of comprehension, and underlying communicative intent" (p. 183). Delayed echolalia has also been referred to as old forms applied to new situations. The language-disordered child has the unique ability to verbally imitate sophisticated linguistic sentences and paragraphs. The echolalic production is often quite deceptive in terms of the child's actual spontaneous ability.

The fact that the child uses old forms in new contexts indicates that on some associative level he or she establishes a relationship between a linguistic form (as rigid as it is) and an event. The production of a delayed echolalic response indicates that the child perceives a relationship between a verbal utterance and a context. As the child's linguistic abilities increase he or she is able to substitute, delete, and/or conjoin elements in the echoed response (i.e., delayed mitigated echolalia). In order to be considered as delayed echolalic utterances, the production had to satisfy one of the following criteria: (1) the repetition had to be beyond the child's syntactic abilities; and/or (2) the utterances had to be rigid and routinized strings. The data indicated that delayed echolalia included utterances that serve different functions, both interactive and noninteractive. A semantic analysis indicates that the echolalic utterance presents a much more sophisticated linguistic ability than do the child's spontaneous productions. Delayed echolalia is not a simplistic or unitary form; it represents a continuum of interaction and comprehension. The authors also indicate that echolalia may vary in its conventionality as a symbolic communicative signal. The listener's interpretation of the echolalic utterance is going to be based on his or her knowledge of the child and characteristics of the shared context.

Language development, production, and creativity depend on an analytic style of processing that offsets the gestalt processing style. In order to generate language, children must learn to use linguistic rules to combine and recombine the basic units. Without a working knowledge of the meaningful units of language, the language-disordered child is doomed to surface associations of long language chunks to contexts. Often the meaning relationship between the memorized chunk and the context is tangential. The discrepancy between form and function presents a serious strain on the communication process. The listener must attempt to derive the child's communicative intent based on what he or she thinks the child means.

Children with language disorders often utilize language patterns that are characterized by repetition of unanalyzed forms. These language chunks may or may not be communicative in nature. This language pattern indicates an inability to use generative rules for production purposes and an inability to analyze the internal structure of another's production. The gestalt and analytic styles represent processing abilities on opposite ends of a continuum. Since the language-disordered child may use an extreme style of gestalt processing, generative language development becomes a very difficult process. "Those who remain primarily echolalic demonstrate a failure to move along the continuum toward analytic processing due to cognitive limitations" (p. 303). It is proposed that as spontaneous utterances increase, echolalia decreases. Spontaneous productions appear to indicate more flexibility in the use of combinatorial rules. This movement toward the analytic end of the processing continuum is necessary for the development of semantic-syntactic relations. In language-disordered children, echolalia may constitute a protracted period of developmental *freeze*. Echolalia represents a phase of development that signals severe limitations in information processing and linguistic comprehension. The amount of time a child remains at this phase is often a cue to the degree of developmental deficit.

As children move along a production-comprehension continuum to a more spontaneous generation of language forms and functions, *word* development may present deficits in vocabulary acquisition and word meaning. During the second and third years of life, children acquire a working vocabulary at a rapid rate. Children who present with semantic deficits may have problems with any or all of the following: semantic functions, categorical skills, vocabulary development, word meaning, relational meaning, determining causes, inferential skills, associations, attributes, narrative schemata, nonliteral meaning, and comprehension skills. Children with semantic problems often have poor comprehension of words and, as a result, poor understanding of multiple meanings. Deficits in word knowledge may become compounded over time, leaving the child with a more limited word base from which he or she cannot further learn to comprehend and to produce spoken language (Nippold, 1992).

Many children with language learning deficits are often late to acquire word knowledge within the lexical system. They are slow to add new words to the system because of pervasive information-processing difficulties. Language-disordered children have significant difficulty in information retrieval as well as in categorical organization, so spontaneous introduction of new information is as difficult as retrieval of old information. Whether there is a problem with information storage and/or retrieval limitations, preschool children with semantic language deficits continue to have severe word-finding difficulties. The deficits in word knowledge ultimately impact on the child's difficulties with learning to read and academic-based instruction.

Semantic Intervention Strategies

Clinical intervention programs need to include goals to develop semantic-syntactic relationships. The child's direct experiences with agents, actions, and objects in social contexts provide knowledge of communicative and semantic functions. Learning must occur in a social situation so that he or she can observe and perform social functions. The mapping of linguistic occurrences onto nonlinguistic ones allows the language-disordered child to extract the internal consistencies that underlie semantic-syntactic relationships in language.

Primary in this specific section is expanding the child's word knowledge and storage to specifically address word-finding problems. Every opportunity must be offered to study new words and to provide instruction on characteristics that will reinforce processing and organization in memory (Nippold, 1992). Part of the development of meaning involves the child's experience in learning about the word. In beginning this process it becomes important to identify common words that have concrete experiences in the child's daily activities.

Focusing on target words through semantic mapping activities provides children with a mechanism to reinforce associations between their activities and the words as well as between associated words. Clearly, such word charting and semantic mapping make the target words salient and relevant to children's personal experiences. The ultimate process is to provide enough word knowledge so that children can develop strategies and cues that are critical for spontaneous word retrieval and usage (Bjork & Bjork, 1992).

Classroom activities that utilize experience-based instruction and have a high degree of routinization increase the child's word-finding predictability. New vocabulary can be introduced in familiar activities and routines. This allows the child the opportunity to learn about how the word is used in relation to other words and within the framework of an action-based activity. Activities that involve matching, categorizing, and sorting enhance conceptual knowledge by focusing on object features or characteristics. The child's lexicon can be analyzed to determine the semantic functions and lexical categories that need to be facilitated in his or her vocabulary. Based on such an analysis, classroom activities can be developed that highlight specific words, content categories, and semantic relations. Telling stories, providing descriptions, and predicting specific outcomes can also facilitate the production side of new word acquisition. The following provides a short description of Jonathan's semantic deficits.

JONATHAN

In the classroom Jonathan demonstrates inconsistent use and knowledge of phases I and II of Bloom and Lahey's content categories. At this time, Jonathan's vocabulary shows limited variety with regard to the use of nouns, verbs, and adjectives. He inconsistently follows one-step directions. Jonathan requires verbal prompts and models to respond to *wh-* questions—who, what, and where. When he responds to questions, his responses are frequently routinized strings of words that are often taken from commercials; his comprehension at times is questionable. Jonathan utilizes a gestalt style of processing, which provides the underpinnings of the echolalic responses that appear as long chunks of information.

Given verbal/visual prompts, Jonathan is able to categorize objects by color, size, shape, and class; however, he demonstrates difficulty with regard to categorizing objects by their function and location. At the present time he cannot describe, define, or elaborate on events or actions. He does not demonstrate inferential skills, attribution, or verbal sequencing. He has difficulty comprehending basic cause-and-effect relationships. His problem-solving skills, verbal and nonverbal, are severely limited.

Semantic Goals

1. To encode a range of semantic functions.
2. To encode semantic relations: action + object, agent + action.
3. To improve ability to follow verbal directions.
4. To encode nouns (objects).
5. To encode verbs (actions).
6. To develop functional vocabulary.
7. To increase spontaneous verbal productions.
8. To respond to simple *wh-* questions.

LANGUAGE FORM

Normal Syntactic Abilities

Syntax appears only when the user discovers that words can be combined in such a way that a certain combination of words actually expresses more than the meaning of any of the individual words. During the third year of life, children begin to encode meaning syntactically in the form of phrases, sentences, and, finally, narratives. In the process of combining words, they learn that words must be organized into sentences following specific linguistic rules and that ideas can be expressed by using sentence structures that express questions, negation, coordination, sequence, causality, and temporality. Conventional forms are important to the expression of ideas. They also expand their conversational abilities. They learn the responsibilities and behaviors related to the differing roles of speaker-initiator and speaker-responder. They can take turns by maintaining a conversational topic for four or five exchanges and can communicatively repair a breakdown in an exchange.

The complexity of a child's language involves a number of components. Sentences are made up of words, clauses, and phrases. As language becomes more complex, the internal structure of the sentence becomes more sophisticated. This means that the sentence gets longer, phrases are developed into noun phrases and verb phrases, and clauses are embedded—one clause functioning as a constituent of another. Children begin to use embedded clauses and can join sentences sometime after thirty-six months. The simple active declarative sentence produced between twenty-four and thirty months is replaced by a complex sentence structure with multiple embeddings by forty-one to forty-eight months of age. In addition to learning to generate complex sentences, children also learn to produce different types of sentence structures: negatives, interrogatives, and imperatives. Each sentence type has its own conceptual basis as well as a specific syntactic structure. Each sentence type reflects the child's ability to manipulate the linguistic structures of his or her language. As the child's conceptual abilities become more complex, more flexible, and more sophisticated, he or she is able to produce more linguistically complex sentence types and sentence forms. Each sentence type—negative, interrogative, and imperative—has an early or primary form, which over time becomes more adult-like in structure.

The most common indicator of sentence length is Mean Length of Utterance (MLU), which is determined by counting the number of meaningful units or morphemes in fifty or one hundred utterances from a child's spontaneous speech sample. The number of units is then divided by the number of utterances recorded. The Mean Length of Utterance is often used as an indicator of language complexity. As children begin to express agent-action-object sequences, they begin to add morphological structures such as modifiers and auxiliaries. Morphological inflections begin to appear around twenty-seven months of age. Brown (1973) identified the sequential acquisition of early morphological structures in children; although the rate of development varies, the order of acquisition remains fairly predictable.

Curtiss (1981) proposed that language components emerge as a function of development of cognitive knowledge. The development of a normal linguistic system in which structure is related to meaning requires an interfacing of linguistic and nonlinguistic cognitive development. Curtiss suggested that lexical and relational semantic abilities are linked to broader conceptual development, but that morphological and syntactic abilities are not. As the child's linguistic structure becomes more sophisticated, his conventional forms begin to approximate those of the adults in his environment. The form and structure become more complex, more embedded, and more independent of the immediate context. Ultimately, children can share information in a series of exchanges during a conversation or they can narrate a sophisticated story script that describes characters, events, a conclusion, and a moral. Ultimately, linguistic structure carries its own forms and it is the structure that supports the meaning; the child learns to manipulate structure for the sake of meaning. The final accomplishment for the normal language user is the acquisition of metalinguistic skills.

Metalinguistic Skills

Metalinguistics represents a new and vital area of child language acquisition. The research in this area has proliferated in the past several years, suggesting that there are many different metas. Production and comprehension skills represent primary abilities in children; when these skills are acquired during the preschool years, the child learns to conceptualize his or her language abilities. Metalinguistic skills represent a higher conceptual understanding of production and comprehension rules. Metalinguistics is the ability to revise, to reflect, and to repair the rules of language. This means that the child not only has normal abilities but also has acquired a conceptual insight about the language rules that he or she is using (Mundy, Sigman, Ungerer, & Sherman, 1987).

The meta ability suggests a level of conceptualization in the language learner that goes beyond learning the rules of language. The ability here suggests that the rules have already been acquired and the child can step back from the process and conceptualize those rules by talking about them. It is almost as though language production and comprehension skills represent primary abilities—a mountain that must be climbed. Once having climbed the mountain and acquired the language foundation, the child stands on top with an ability to look around at all of the rules that he has mastered. He is aware of a process and he can make judgments about the integrity of the language experience. He has the ability to reflect upon his knowledge of language; he can talk about his language experience.

Another analogy might be a child learning to play tennis. Understanding how to hold the racket, how to swing the racket, how to stand, how to serve, where to hit the ball, how many games to the set, how many sets to the match—once the child has learned all of these things and has played the game, she can often step back and talk about the game as a whole. In the case of language learning, the child has acquired the pragmatic, semantic, syntactic, and phonological abilities that all become integrated and used at the same time. With this acquisition the language learner can take a step back and understand that there are language rules; she can talk about the language rules and ask questions about them. This insight, this conceptual understanding that she is talking about a rule, indicates that the child has a metalinguistic skill. She is aware of language structures and can make judgments about the integrity of her or someone else's production. The preschool child can make judgments about the acceptability of someone else's utterances and can also repair the structural aspects at the sound, word, and sentence level.

Metalinguistic abilities usually develop after a preschool child has mastered a linguistic structure. Metalinguistics involves the ability of the child to conceptualize his knowledge of the rules of his language: talking about talking, talking about thinking, and thinking about talking. The meta is a level of conceptual development that includes metapragmatic, metacognition, metahumor, and metacomprehension skills. With metacognitive skills, the child has the ability to deal abstractly with his own thought processes in comprehension, memory, information processing, reasoning, and problem solving (Brown, 1978). Deficits in language production and comprehension obviously interfere with the development of these more abstract meta skills.

The Language-Disordered Child

With pervasive problems in broader conceptual areas, it is not surprising that a child with a language disorder presents with deficits in morphological and syntactic structures. Grammatical morphemes and function words are often omitted; speech may be telegraphic, simplistic, and structurally restricted. Bartolucci, Pierce, Streiner, and Eppel (1976) described difficulty with the

developmental use of verb endings, such as past tense and pres
These researchers did not interpret the findings as a difficulty w
cal structure per se, but rather as a difficulty with semantic deve
appears that the more basic problem for language-disordered childre
they do not understand the underlying conceptual ideas, such as past
rence, that contribute to the formulation of language. In addition, they h
difficulties using or manipulating specific linguistic forms of language becau
they do not understand their semantic counterparts. It seems that the syntactic delays and limitations are related to general developmental delays; there is an underlying difficulty in the child's understanding of language as a system.

Metadeficits

Children with language disorders do not develop intact production and comprehension skills. They do not acquire complex sentence structures or the variety of sentence types; very often their sentences are simple in structure with many morphological errors or omissions. They have difficulty integrating meaning with structure in language. As a result, when syntactic complexity should increase, the syntactic structures utilized for production purposes remain simple. Often these children remain unaware that there is a breakdown in the communicative process or a linguistic error produced by another speaker. Kamhi (1987) notes that even when they have the ability to comprehend or produce a structure, it does not ensure that they will have the ability to judge the appropriate use of that structure in another speaker's language.

Kamhi writes that the linguistic deficits that are characteristic of language-disordered children serve to explain some of the metalinguistic problems in development. They have more difficulty than children with typical language abilities in making judgments and revising syntactic forms. Kamhi suggests that they acquire these forms much later than most children, and, as a result, they have much less time to utilize and conceptualize them. They also have difficulty acquiring grammatical forms such as auxiliaries, inflections, pronouns, and conjunctions. These language forms prove to be particularly difficult to symbolically represent because they do not have a concrete referent. In addition, Johnston and Wiesmer (1983) indicate that language-disordered children have difficulty in coding the nonlinguistic aspects of language. As a result, the semantic-conceptual foundation does not provide a strong base for linguistic development.

Syntactic Intervention Strategies

Perhaps the most significant issue in the facilitation of the structural aspects of language involves ensuring the underlying comprehension strategies. Specifically, training children to parrot form without function is not a clinically sound strategy. It is important to develop linguistic structures within a communication framework. Otherwise, the language-disordered child will not acquire the

her knowledge to other situations, contexts, and language
at to teach a child it is reasonable to follow a developmen-
onsider what is relevant as well as meaningful given the
nvironment. One must take into consideration the child's
nd personal needs in deciding on structures that should
ech/language pathologist needs to survey all of the pro-
ofessionals working with the language-disordered child.
echanism to develop and cross-reference activities with

Bunce, Ruder, and Ruder (1985) describe the use of a miniature linguistic system (MLS) that can be used to facilitate the acquisition of syntactic structures. Children receive specific training on verb-object constructions, with attention to word order in training and generalization to untrained structures. A single verb can be paired with a variety of nouns to expand the child's conceptual understanding of the action word: *push car, push truck, push chair,* etc. This results in a matrix that develops a range of semantic-syntactic associations. Once the child has learned a number of verb-object communications, subjects can be added to generate S-V-O constructions: *Mommy push car, Daddy push truck,* and so on.

Syntactic training should focus on utilizing multiple exemplars to provide a mechanism for generalization to untrained semantic-syntactic constructions. Different objects from the same class of objects (such as different cars) should be used to reinforce the child's conceptualization of linguistic forms representing a category rather than a specific referent. Holding the verb constant and changing objects can be alternated with holding the object constant and alternating verbs. Alternating and contrasting specific syntactic forms reinforces the semantic-conceptual changes in meaning: *Mommy push car* results in a very different environmental event than *Mommy push chair.* This also allows the child to observe the result of her linguistic production. Environmental consequences serve to enhance the relationship between linguistic and nonlinguistic occurrences.

Language facilitation can be accomplished most effectively in the child's natural environment. If the language structures are not relevant to the child, he will not use them. It is important to note as well that if the language structures are not meaningful to teachers and caretakers, they will not use them. Language training will only generalize if everyone contributes to the process and has an investment in the child's success. Facilitators need to be involved with the development of programming and need to be monitored on how the program is being used in daily activities.

The focus of training must shift from language form to language use. In the real world, the child's ability to function on the job—in a vocational setting or in a restaurant—is more important than specific forms or specific structures of language. It appears that language skills involving social behaviors such as interpersonal abilities, politeness, conversational skills, following directions, and self-control are rated as being much more important than the production of sophisticated sentences. It is critical, therefore, to recognize when language form training must be replaced by the more practical communication skills; in this way we recognize that the language-disordered child must learn to function within the realities of his or her social context and environment.

JONATHAN

At this time Jonathan's syntactic structures consist of echolalic utterances and his spontaneous Mean Length of Utterance (MLU) has been calculated to be less than 1.0. He displays significant difficulty in integrating the linguistic components of form, content, and use. He also displays difficulty linking ideas to their appropriate linguistic form and channeling those formats into cohesive sequential sentence structures. Consequently, due to conceptual problems in language, Jonathan does not use his language creatively. As the level of linguistic complexity and demand increases, linguistic organizational problems become more evident, thereby affecting his ability to function as an effective communicator.

Jonathan requires a multimodal approach to learning (i.e., auditory, visual, tactile, kinesthetic). He displays difficulty consistently responding to auditory stimuli presented at the level of conversational speech. These difficulties do not appear to be a problem of audition, but rather a problem involving language processing. Jonathan relies on routinized linguistic forms, verbal models, and physical prompts in order to be an effective communicator. This gives rise to problems involving responding, regulating, and demonstrating a creative use of language. Therefore, he experiences significant social and linguistic difficulties when presented with a more sophisticated group of language users. In socially oriented situations, Jonathan does not exhibit the metalinguistic skills that would indicate an ability to revise, to reflect, and to repair his language or the language productions of others.

Goals

1. To increase spontaneous language production.
2. To encode semantic-syntactic relations: agent + action + object.
3. To encode simple *wh-* questions.

SUMMARY

This chapter provided a profile on language-disordered children. The characteristics described are not exhaustive nor are they presented to suggest that all language-disordered children evidence all of the characteristics discussed. The profile presents a philosophical approach to educational programming. It underscores the need to utilize a variable in education—language rather than label, IQ, and/or behavior. It is the position of the authors that although children share many different learning problems, they all share one common problem as children with developmental disorders—they all have language-learning deficits. It becomes rather intriguing to determine how the profiles vary from one language-disordered child to another, but over time it has become clear that there are more similarities among language-disordered children than there are differences.

Language provides an insight into children and the educational process that has not been a variable before, since other characteristics have been utilized and emphasized. This chapter proposes that children can be identified, classified, and ultimately educated by understanding and addressing specific language-learning needs. Without a doubt, Bloom and Lahey's (1978) commentary on the noncategorical approach to education remains true today. In order to look at children in terms of their language deficits rather than their labels, the educational system itself must be changed. This is a challenge for the future.

In the following chapters of this text, we will discuss various problems in special education, such as early intervention, testing and assessment, family issues, the role of the parent, advocacy, and the classroom laboratory. Language provides a mechanism for us as educators to reorganize and restructure educational instruction. It is clearly a powerful tool that provides for a taxonomy in educational philosophy that has not been adequately utilized before. Another challenge, however, is that academic-based instruction at the university level must also be changed.

This text proposes a set of ideas, techniques, and beliefs that are very different from the way in which most educators work and think. The question becomes: Who will use this book? The answer is the academician, the teacher, the educator, and the specialist who believe that education needs to be infused with a new viewpoint. Clearly, this text is not going to answer every question for every educator, but it will focus everyone's attention on an immediate issue—all developmentally disabled children have a language-communication disorder. The severity of the disorder may vary; some of the characteristics of the disorder may vary; some of the related problems may vary—but the language learning deficit is *the problem.* Heretofore, the language deficit has been a sideline issue, a related issue. This text suggests that the language disorder must be the central issue in understanding these children, their learning needs, and ultimately the educational programming required to meet those needs. It is my personal belief that the text will encourage thoughtful consideration and the formulation of probing questions in our professional discipline.

A FEW WORDS FROM TOYA DAVIS

My name is Toya Davis. I am the parent of a handicapped child. When Dr. Tiegerman asked me to share my experiences I spent a great deal of time thinking about what would be meaningful to students and professionals reading this book. Perhaps the most important thing that I can share about Jonathan is that he is a language-disordered child. Frankly, ten years ago when my son entered SLCD (School for Language and Communication Development) as a three-year-old, I had no understanding of what that meant. My family thought that Jonathan was lazy. My husband thought that Jonathan was a late talker. My pediatrician thought that there was something wrong but he did not understand that Jonathan's problem was more than just learning to say words. Learning about language has been an incredible experience for me. As a parent, I feel that a world of knowledge has been opened to me through parent training and through my son's experience. When I read now that language is a symbolic representational system I can truly say that I know what that means for my son. In learning about language I have learned about reading, socialization, verbal math problems, and storytelling. I have learned how to apply all of my language knowledge to other related areas in Jonathan's education.

I have often been told as a parent advocate in school districts that the problem with SLCD is that all it teaches "is language; it does not teach anything else." This statement has always amused me since I know *now* that there is nothing else. Without language my child could not have functioned in school. Without language as a strong foundation to learning, my Jonathan could never have been mainstreamed into a regular class or program. Learning about language is learning about yourself and the system that allows you to develop into other areas, such as reading. Language allows you to talk about yourself, to talk about what you think and what you feel. I have come to understand as a parent that if my child does not have language he has nothing—he has silence. When I read the original chapter for this book I cried. I know how important it is as a parent of a language-disordered child for teachers, specialists, and special educators to understand who my son is. My Jonathan, like so many other children, is language disordered. Jonathan needs to be recognized; his problem needs to be recognized. Parents and professionals need to understand the road that I have traveled as a parent of a handicapped child and the road that my son has traveled in learning language.

REFERENCES

ASHA Committee on Language, Speech and Hearing Services in the Schools. (April 1980). Definitions for communicative disorders and differences. *ASHA, 22,* 317–318.

Bartolucci, G., Pierce, S., Streiner, D., & Eppel, P. T. (1976). Phonological investigation of verbal autistic and mentally retarded subjects. *Journal of Autism and Childhood Schizophrenia, 6,* 303–316.

Bates, E., Benigni, L., Bretherton, I., Camaioni, L., & Volterra, V. (1979). *The emergence of symbols: Cognition and communication in infancy.* New York: Academic Press.

Beisler, J., & Tsai, L. (1983). A pragmatic approach to increase expressive language skills in young autistic children. *Journal of Autism and Developmental Disorders, 13,* 287–303.

Bernard-Opitz, V. (1982). Pragmatic analysis of the communicative disorder of an autistic child. *Journal of Speech and Hearing Disorders, 47,* 99–109.

Bjork, R. A., & Bjork, E. L. (1992). A new theory of disuse and an old theory of stimulus fluctuation. In A. F. Healy, S. M. Kosslyn, & R. M. Shiffrin (Eds.), *From learning processes to cognitive processes: Essays in honor of William K. Estes* (Vol. 2, pp. 35–67). Hillsdale, NJ: Erlbaum.

Bloom, L., & Lahey, M. (1978). *Language development and language disorders.* New York: Wiley.

Bowerman, M. (1978). The acquisition of word meaning: An investigation in some current conflicts. In N. Waterson & C. Snow (Eds.), *The development of communication.* New York: Wiley.

Brown, A. L. (1978). Knowing when, where and how to remember a problem of metacognition. In R. Glaser (Ed.), *Advances in instructional psychology.* Hillsdale, NJ: Erlbaum.

Brown, R. (1973). *A first language: The early stages.* Cambridge: Harvard University Press.

Bunce, B. H., Ruder, K., & Ruder, C. (1985). Using a miniature linguistic system in teaching syntax: Two case studies. *Journal of Speech and Hearing Disorders, 50,* 247–253.

Clark, E. (1973). What's in a word? On the child's acquisition of semantics in his first language. In T. E. Moore (Ed.), *Cognitive development and the acquisition of language* (pp. 65–110). New York: Academic Press.

Curtiss, S. (1981). Dissociations between language and cognition: Cases and implications. *Journal of Autism and Developmental Disorders, 11,* 15–30.

Duchan, J. (1986). Learning to describe events. *Topics in Language Disorders, 6,* 27–36.

Fay, W. (1967). Mitigated echolalia of children. *Journal of Speech and Hearing Research, 10,* 305–310.

Hubbell, R. (1981). *Children's language disorders: An integrated approach.* Englewood Cliffs, NJ: Prentice-Hall.

Johnston, J., & Wiesmer, S. (1983). Mental rotation abilities in language disordered children. *Journal of Speech and Hearing Research, 26,* 397–404.

Kamhi, A. G. (1987). Mental abilities in language impaired children. *Topics in Language Disorders, 7,* 1–12.

Kintsch, W. (1974). *The representation of meaning in memory.* Hillsdale, NJ: Erlbaum.

Mundy, P., Sigman, M., Ungerer, J., & Sherman, T. (1987). Nonverbal communication and play correlates of language development in autistic children. *Journal of Autism and Developmental Disorders, 17,* 349–364.

Nelson, K. (1974). Concept, word and sentence: Inter-relations in acquisition and development. *Psychological Review, 81,* 267–285.

Nippold, M. (1992). The nature of normal and disordered word finding in children and adolescents. *Topics in Language Disorders, 13,* 1–14.

Prizant, B., & Duchan, J. (1981). The functions of immediate echolalia in autistic children. *Journal of Speech and Hearing Disorders, 46,* 241–249.

Prizant, B., & Rydell, P. (1984). Analysis of functions of delayed echolalia in autistic children. *Journal of Speech and Hearing Research 27,* 183–192.

Prizant, B. M., & Wetherby, A. M. (1987). Communicative intent: A framework for understanding social-communicative behavior in autism. *Journal of the American Academy of Child and Adolescent Psychiatry, 26,* 472–479.

Prizant, B., & Wetherby, A. M. (1990). Toward an integrated view of early language and communication development and socio-emotional development. *Topics in Language Disorders, 10,* 1–16.

Wetherby, A. M. (1986). Ontogeny of communicative functions in autism. *Journal of Autism and Developmental Disorders, 16,* 295–316.

Yoshinaga-Itano, C., & Downey, D. (1986). A hearing impaired child's acquisition of schemata: Something's missing. *Topics in Language Disorders, 7,* 45–57.

CHAPTER

2

THE CHANGING ROLE OF THE FAMILY

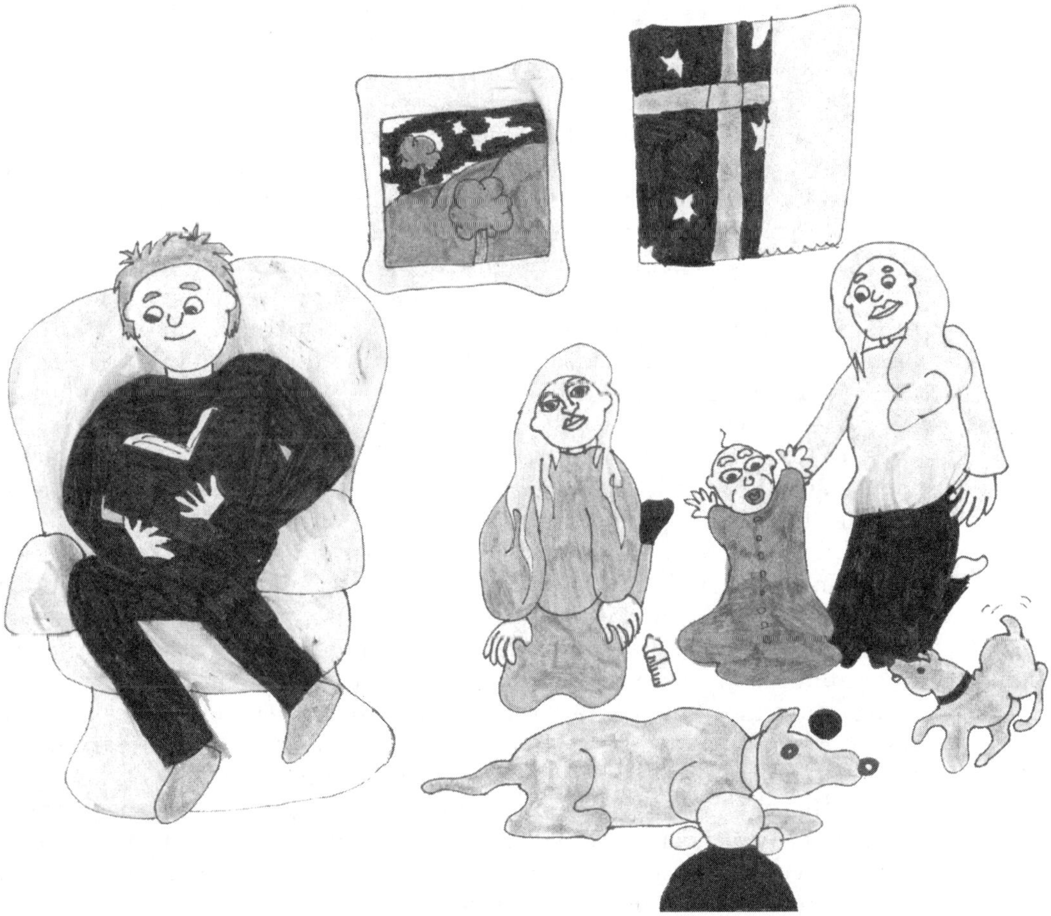

Historically, education has been left to the educators. The separation of school and home in education can only be likened to the fundamental separation of church and state. After the struggle is over and advocacy results in change, parents are relegated to the home rather than offered a place in the classroom. Few schools in the United States provide formalized parent-education classes and even fewer integrate the parent into the educational process as an equal partner in decision making. Parents are not viewed separately from their children. Parents of children with disabilities are often seen through their children. They are perceived as being the same as their children, and, in addition, are seen as having different needs from those of parents of typical children without disabilities. The reality is that all parents share common needs and goals in the educational process.

The purpose of this chapter is to discuss the complex educational issues that face families of disabled children in a multicultural environment. Families are now addressing the identification of children with disabilities at a much earlier stage of development. The structure of the family has changed in the past several decades; it is complicated further by the demands of multicultural problems, such as cultural diversity, language differences, and poverty, which are ultimately the critical issues that affect disabled preschool children, as well as their educational programming. The school can no longer view children separately from their families. Language-disordered preschool children must be evaluated, educated, and understood in terms of the ecology of their families; these children's problems are a mirror reflection of dynamic family issues that must be considered along with special education goals.

A family assessment should highlight the strengths and weaknesses of the child's primary environment and primary agents for change. The school can never replace the home in the life of any child, particularly not in the life of the language-disordered preschool child. Given the demands of the multicultural family, the school needs to empower, to educate, and to mobilize the family for everyone's success.

Since families enter the system for the first time with the preschool child, their insights, their attitudes, and their beliefs provide instruction for all of us as educators. In preparation for this chapter, parents from all over the Long Island, New York, community were polled through questionnaires. The cultural, linguistic, and economic diversity of the families polled represent a wide range of statements and comments. Since this is a chapter on families, a great deal of time and effort went into developing and evaluating the questionnaires. Four hundred questionnaires were disseminated; 325 were collected and analyzed. The chapter organization makes a commitment to families by printing their personal viewpoints. Perhaps the greatest opportunity for learning comes from listening; in this case, listening to the voices of parents. Again, the purpose of this chapter is to present a number of issues that affect the parents and families of preschool children with language disorders, and to highlight the importance of an ecological approach to understanding the diverse multicultural needs of families in education.

Public Law 99-457 has mandated the development of early intervention programs for disabled preschool children. The development of early intervention programs has raised a number of issues about the educational process (Krauss, 1990). This chapter will include discussion of a number of critical issues in early intervention:

- Children must be educated along with their families
- Parents must be trained to function as child facilitators
- Parents must be incorporated in the decision-making process
- Parents must be viewed as the child's lifelong advocates
- Traditional education must change to a family-centered approach

The knowledge base for parent education has been developed from research investigations of children with disabilities and their families during the past three decades.

Research studies have stressed the importance of training parents as facilitators to generalize goals to contexts outside the classroom (Bronfenbrenner, 1977; McDade & Varnedoe, 1987). The results of such investigations have not affected the plight of parents of nondisabled children, nor have they been incorporated into most educational programs for children with disabilities. Although it is clear that educational development of children with disabilities can be enhanced if parents reinforce classroom goals at home, few schools provide parents with formal academic instruction in areas such as language development, language disorders, psychosocial development, behavioral management, and intervention techniques.

As far as federal and state regulations are concerned, parent training and education are recommended, but not mandated, services. Parent-training goals are rarely if ever a part of the child's Individualized Educational Plan (IEP). Therefore, it should not be surprising that even less attention is paid to parents of nondisabled children in educational settings. How often do parents sit in the classroom to observe their children's learning or the educational process? How often do parents receive formal instruction so that they can teach their children reading or math at home? How do parents learn what teachers know about the educational process? Given the state of education in the United States, can parents continue to leave education to teachers? They are going to have to advocate for educational services for *themselves,* along with services for their children. They are going to have to advocate for educational recognition and inclusion in the process.

Research investigations in the area of child language development have focused on the nature of maternal input and mother-child interaction (Cross, 1977; Kaiser & Blair, 1987; Tiegerman & Siperstein, 1984). Such studies point out the role of the parent and the home context in early child development. Unfortunately most parents do not read professional journals, but the message is being transmitted to and translated for them in trade books such as

Babysignals (Lynch-Fraser & Tiegerman, 1987). The new message stresses that since education begins well before children enter school and continues throughout adulthood, parents need to establish an early long-term relationship with the educational system and process. This new philosophy needs to be reflected in the educational system and process.

THE FAMILY AND THE EDUCATION MODEL

The traditional model of education presents a number of basic assumptions about the professional-parent relationship. The traditional model of intervention is based on an educational system that has been in place since 1975 and the passage of Public Law 94-142 (Education of All Handicapped Children Act). In this traditional model the first assumption involves special education.

Special Education

In the United States, special education facilitators have been the primary teachers who provide service for children with disabilities. States have different teaching certifications that are either specific in nature (teacher of the mentally retarded, teacher of the autistic, teacher of the learning disabled) or general in nature (teacher of special education) and cover all disabled populations. Whatever the certification, special education over the past several decades has become highly specialized and separated from mainstream or regular education. The philosophical notion or underlying premise of special education is that the developmentally disabled child requires not only different instruction but also highly specialized educational curricula. As a result of this approach to the special-needs child, special education programming has proliferated in terms of the number of programs developed and the number of children served since 1975. It is important to know that prior to 1975, children with developmental disabilities were warehoused and did not receive specialized programming in public school facilities (Yell & Espin, 1990). In 1986, the pendulum began to swing in the opposite direction.

Terms such as *segregation* and *Regular Education Initiative* (REI) have been used to publicize the issue of separate special education programs. Since developmentally disabled children present with highly idiosyncratic learning dynamics, they have been placed in specialized classrooms with other developmentally disabled children. The terms *mainstreaming* and *REI* have become quite confusing due to the volatility of the segregation issue. Madeline Wills, Under Secretary of the U.S. Department of Education, forcefully advocated for a change in the way in which special-needs children are educated in public schools. The notion proposed in the late 1980s stressed that children with developmental disabilities should not be placed in segregated (separate) settings, classrooms, or schools. Many states moving in this direction have encouraged the placement of children with developmental disabilities in regular education classrooms (REI) in order for them to experience "normalization" in learning (Yanok, 1986). The use of the term *segregated* with disabled children suggests that the change from specialization to regularization is based on political issues and not necessarily on educational research. There are two basic questions that still need to be addressed before this movement in regularization progresses too far. Experimental research needs to answer the following questions:

1. Will the disabled child benefit educationally from a placement in a regular class (with nondisabled children)? How should the term *benefit* be defined across populations of children?
   a. Will children with developmental disabilities who have different disability labels benefit from placement in regular classes (with nondisabled children)?
   b. Will children with developmental disabilities who have different levels of severity (in functioning) benefit from placement in regular classes (with nondisabled children)?
2. How will the placement of children with developmental disabilities in regular education classes impact (either positively or negatively) the educational advancement of the nondisabled children in those classes?

In the special education classroom, the hours of educational instruction remain 9:00 A.M. to 3:00 P.M. If there is a question about changing special edu cation, perhaps this area also needs to be addressed. Since the requirements for special-education children are quite different than those for nondisabled children and the needs are much greater, perhaps the hours of instruction should be extended. In addition, the traditional model suggests that the classroom is the primary context for learning. Given the diverse needs of children with developmental disabilities, perhaps either there should be a different focus for learning (i.e., the home or a vocational center) or there should be multiple centers for learning outside of the school. Perhaps one of the critical issues with the special-education child involves "fitting the child to the program" rather than "fitting the program to the child." The child with developmental disabilities is *not* a slow learner or a younger typical child. The special-needs child is a different learner who requires not just quantitative but qualitative differences in programming. How can education continue to meet the language-disordered preschool child's individual needs without compromising the LRE process?

Least Restrictive Environment

In dealing with language-disordered preschool children there should always be a focus on developmental and educational needs. The educational model is one that provides services for children during the traditional hours with teachers and therapists. The passage of PL 94-142 mandated a free and appropriate public education. The resulting interpretation, along with the regular education initiative (REI), is that the least restrictive environment (LRE) is the regular classroom, which mixes disabled and nondisabled children. Since the passage of PL 94-142, children with disabilities have been "fit" into the traditional educational model and classroom. The assumption has been that the opportunity for interaction with nondisabled children was not only beneficial but also educationally sound. The reality, however, is that the declassification process from most restrictive to least restrictive must be a gradual process based on the readiness of the disabled child.

There is nothing magical about placing children with disabilities in a normalized environment with nondisabled children. The question remains—is the child with disabilities ready for this experience? Will the child with disabilities benefit from interaction with normal children in a classroom? Have educators really left the education of children with disabilities to typical children and the chance for some social interaction? Can a chance encounter substitute for a regulated therapeutic environment? The regular education initiative does not appear to be an educational fad; it does not portend well for children with disabilities if educational decisions are based on anything but individual child needs. Finally, fitting the language-disordered preschool child into the traditional model would perhaps be more acceptable if there were not so many serious problems in educating nondisabled children from culturally diverse backgrounds (Vohs, 1989). It is clearly time to change our focus from traditional educational models to the development of alternative systems and programs to meet the specific needs of preschool children with disabilities and their multicultural families (Yoshida, Fenton, Kaufman, & Maxwell, 1978). In fact, parents who have been trained as teachers and facilitators may be education's answer to the transition process from the self-contained classroom placement to the regular education classroom.

The Family as Ecological System

The assessment of family needs and of the child with disabilities in relation to those needs underscores the interactive influences of the child on the family and the family on the child (Sameroff & Chandler, 1975). There are many stresses in the family of the child with disabilities. Parents need to go through a "passages" process; they must progress through stages of reality and acceptance in ultimately understanding the needs of the child. In the framework of the family, the child's development and progress can be assessed in terms of the proactive involvement of family members (Dunst, 1985).

The classroom cannot replace the home and teachers cannot replace parents. Educational success is clearly dependent on the empowerment of the family. In this model, teachers and parents must share in the responsibilities related to understanding and educating the disabled child. Dunst's Proactive Empowerment through Partnerships (PEP) (Dunst, 1985) shifts decision making from the professional to the parents. It becomes the role of the teacher to facilitate parent-child learning by empowering parents with knowledge. Parents are given the skills and competencies to access resources in the educational system and the community to meet family needs. This shift of control and decision making from professionals to parents highlights the fact that a teacher's involvement with a disabled child is for a relatively short time. Parents, on the other hand, do not change at the end of every school year; they are involved for a lifetime.

The knowledgeable family is the independent family that advocates effectively for the child and understands his or her internal strengths. Bronfenbrenner's (1977) ecological model focuses on the family and its external network to assess the nature of the support to the family since the child can be positively or negatively affected by the family's reaction to these environmental factors:

1. The child with disabilities impacts the emotional and social development of individual family members as well as the family as an interactive unit. The family must learn to understand the child's role in the family (see Figure 2-1).
2. Educational changes in the child with disabilities will affect the family. It is important to facilitate the family's active involvement with and understanding of such changes. The process of change is difficult and an understanding of the family as a unit will help teachers realize the impact of child changes on the family's adaptive abilities.
3. Empowering parents involves them in educational decision making and develops their role in the process.
4. The internal growth and emotional actualization of the family will facilitate the development of family goals rather than child goals. The family must learn to see the disabled child as a member of the group.

The Family and the School

The National Association of School Psychologists (Barona & Garcia, 1990) provides the following trends for preschool children:

1. Twenty-four percent of preschool children currently live below the poverty line.
2. One-third of preschool children are nonwhite. By the turn of the century, 40 percent of all children in the United States under six years of age will be nonwhite.
3. By the year 2000, almost 40 percent of all preschool children in the United States will speak a language other than English.

Figure 2-1
How Does the Disabled Child Affect the Family?

. . . The family is affected because with a disabled child comes *lots* of stress. Knowing to love the child yet not spoil him. It's very difficult to know when *not* to feel sorry.

. . . Steven requires a lot more attention than my other two. The attention is divided 30%, 30%, 40%. They accept this.

. . . In the case of a communication deficit, behavior problems can arise. Oftentimes treatment at home may be biased toward the disabled child, which affects the balance of the whole family system.

. . . Ben's language disorder gave rise to frustration on his part when he could not communicate his needs. Older siblings sometimes lose patience with him. They often ignore him like other children.

. . . The child needs extra attention that causes tension with other siblings. In most families *everyone* is very concerned with the child's health and educational progress.

. . . Other siblings try to help the disabled child, sometimes meeting with frustration that leads to anger. The environment can change often. That is upsetting and depressing.

. . . I experience personal frustration due to lack of receptiveness of my child when I talk to him.

. . . I feel anxiety and stress with concern about if he will ever mature and grow to be a happy successful individual and fit into "mainstream society."

. . .The disability can frustrate other family members and can be generally disruptive.

. . . There are good and bad ways it has affected our family. We are all a lot more tolerant of other people's shortcomings. I feel my boys will be better people for having learning problems and in the process of overcoming them will become strong worthwhile adults.

. . . It makes it difficult to do "normal" family things. The disabled child is usually left out.

. . . In different ways. Personally, I think more patience and understanding is involved. Turning a deaf ear to the comments "well-meaning" people say. Being a close family helps everyone deal with it better.

. . . He might need more attention than other family members. Also, it can make it difficult, at times, when interacting with other families who have children.

. . . All people in the family affect the family. When everyone's needs are considered, a family is a cohesive unit. What binds one family together is always different from what binds another, but that they are together is most important.

. . . You are grateful for "little" things that "normal families" take for granted. You pray more and work harder at everything. You are forced to deal with apathy and ignorance from those not aware of the changes a family goes through having a disabled child.

. . . They have been numerous with our family, aside from a calendar always filled with doctor appointments. The sibling jealousy of why Steven gets all the attention is an ongoing battle. Separation of mother and father's time and family during hospital stays. The financial burden of high medical bills has resulted in me going back to work full time. It requires us to be more responsive to Steven at the expense of his sisters and family in general.

4. Eighteen percent of the preschool population was born out of wedlock. It is estimated that 21 percent of those girls will become pregnant in their teens.
5. Almost 45 percent of preschool children will be raised by single parents before they reach the age of eighteen; half will experience one or more family breakups.

6. Fifty-five percent of preschool children currently have mothers who work outside the home. By 1995, 75 percent of their mothers will work outside the home, most in a full-time capacity.

These statistics stress the fact that the traditional family has changed and that there are significant numbers of preschool children who are at risk, who are a minority, who are multicultural, and who come from impoverished backgrounds. The statistical trends are alarming because they highlight the dramatic needs of schools to change their programming to reflect multicultural issues. The educational system, as it is designed from a content and a procedural prospective, cannot possibly meet the complex needs of a multicultural community. Miranda and Santos de Barona (1990) indicate that "the public school system in the United States has not provided children with the skills necessary for success. Particularly at risk are ethnic minorities and children from disadvantaged backgrounds. Educational limitations include lack of appropriate personnel, financial difficulties, and organization hierarchies [that do not] meet the needs of the community environment." The educational literature includes reports of the minority child at risk in the educational system. Whereas early literature attributed the child's failure to the family environment, later literature recognized the role of the educational system in inhibiting the academic progress of minority children, particularly in large urban environments.

The National Commission on Excellence in Education, in its celebrated report, *A Nation at Risk,* indicated the special needs and concerns of ethnic minorities (1983). It also described that parents of minority children find it difficult to advocate for their children's needs, often are naive about the educational setting and special education programs, feel uncomfortable visiting their children's schools, and participate in school activities only to a limited extent when compared to parents generally. The report attributes this lack of parental involvement to the time that activities are scheduled in school, the lack of child care, and the long distances between home and school.

Edwards (1990) indicates that many minority parents do not help their children with homework, not due to lack of concern, but because of their limited English proficiency and their lack of educational skills. Minority families are particularly concerned about the placement of children in bilingual programs. Edwards also indicates that minority parents do not trust the schools their children attend; they believe that there is a general expectation that minority students will perform poorly in school. A significant problem here is the lack of bilingual professionals and teachers in particular who can adequately address the language, communication, and cultural barriers that presently exist. Staff training must be developed and established as a primary goal in the schools, since the multicultural family will represent such a large diverse group in the next decade.

Minority families describe prejudice, language barriers, and cultural difficulties that contribute to school failure and professional reluctance to understand the cultural differences. Families are concerned about getting a quality and relevant education for their children. They want an educational system that reflects their values and cultural prospectives. Minority families feel left out of the educational decision-making process. Edwards (1987) indicated that "parents want to be apprised about specific learning strategies and approaches that they can utilize at home; parents want more information about their children's educational programs and progress." It appears that the families who require the greatest amount of support and who want most to be involved with the educational system are not. What are the barriers that interfere with parental involvement? The subcommittee indicated that parents from minority groups are affected by poor literacy skills, language differences, learning deficits, the inability to understand school personnel and procedures, cultural and physical distance between the school and the community, inability to attend school meetings, and inability to help their children achieve their potentials. Edmonds (1983) argued that "the fact that many poor and minority children fail to master the school curriculum does not reflect deficiencies in the children, but rather inadequacies in the schools themselves" (Neisser, 1986, p. 223).

Brady (1977) indicated that "parent involvement was so critical to the educational process that it should be required," but he cautioned that schools still need to respect individual and cultural differences. They need to develop a central philosophy that translates into program goals and provides the framework for decision making. Parents need to know and to understand the school's operating principles. Part of the educational process should focus on the orientation of parents to the school environment (Bailey & Simeonsson, 1988). Parents should be fully versed in:

a. evaluation procedures and tests
b. the results of all tests, and their child's language, social, and cognitive levels of functioning
c. how children are placed in various classes
d. the developmental characteristics of children in their child's class and in other classes
e. educational goals for the child and the classroom
f. the types of related services and why they are necessary to the development of the child
g. the child's schedule during the week
h. educational timelines during the year for the IEPs, midyear reports, and end-of-year summaries
i. procedures for changing classrooms and services so that they will not feel that decisions concerning children are made arbitrarily

EARLY FAMILY ASSESSMENT

The traditional education system views the disabled child separately from his or her family. The child's developmental difficulties are evaluated by professionals who rarely interview or assess the family as a unit. Assessment procedures should view the child in relation to the family (Bailey, 1991). The evaluation of the child does not include parent-child interactional variables. The entire present evaluation process can be completed by a speech/language pathologist, a psychologist, a social worker, a special education teacher, and a dance-movement therapist with the child alone—without seeing the child and the parents together or the child in the home environment with the family. Figure 2-2 proposes that a family assessment be completed by means of a more natural approach. The evaluation of the child includes an analysis of family interactional variables with parents and siblings in a life center—a simulated home setting—rather than in a traditional therapy room. This would enable the family to interact with one another in a context similar to the home process and experience. The setting itself would readily provide access to interactional variables difficult to assess with traditional assessment tools. The life center would allow families to engage in activities that occur at home while the entire multidisciplinary team has the opportunity to observe. This would also allow parents to observe each other and professionals interacting with the child. Here cross observation stabilizes the evaluation process and its results. Everyone has shared observations with the opportunity for shared perceptions based on those observations.

When parents are involved with diagnostic procedures and the assessment process, they are more accepting of the evaluation results. In addition, when they are given the opportunity to contribute to educational decisions and programming goals, they become more involved with the process of education (Brinckerhoff & Vincent, 1986). A problem that arises from traditional evaluation and diagnostic methodology is that although parents have their own pri-

Figure 2-2
Family Assessment Process

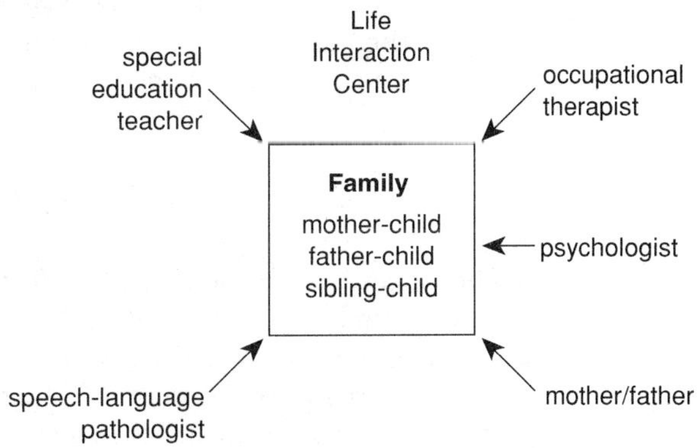

orities concerning the education of the child, when they are not part of the evaluation process, they cannot provide their input to evaluators. The notion that parents cannot be realistic or objective about their child's developmental needs is often used to argue against including them in the process. Sexton, Miller, and Rotatori (1985) indicate that parents can be reliable sources of information that should supplement direct testing and observational techniques. The result of not including them is that the diagnostic team is generating recommendations and goals for a child based on isolated information from a single meeting in an unnatural context.

Fuchs, Fuchs, Power, and Dailey (1985) found that nondisabled children scored similarly when tested by either familiar or unfamiliar examiners, while children with disabilities scored lower with unfamiliar examiners. The traditional diagnostic team is not provided with the time to interact with the child and the family to counteract the possible effect of such professional-child variables. Is it any wonder that parents cannot agree with and accept decisions that they did not help generate? Parents must become members of the diagnostic team and participate in the process if effective family assessment is to be achieved.

1. The disabled child needs to be evaluated by a multidisciplinary team with the parents as members of the team.
2. Professionals should use a range of multicultural assessment instruments, but only after the child has been in an experimental/diagnostic classroom for several weeks and has had multiple opportunities to interact with members of the evaluation team, including the parents.
3. There should be multiple observations of the child in the classroom by the diagnostic team as a group. Group observational analysis and discussion will facilitate a product that reinforces common goals across discipline areas. In the school setting, the classroom represents the most natural context.
4. Parent-child analyses should be part of the diagnostic protocol. The diagnostic team should observe the child in the home with the family, enabling the team to acquire information for a family assessment, as well as information on the quantity and quality of family-child interactions.

Parental Involvement

The parent education process *begins* when the child is initially evaluated to determine his or her candidacy for early intervention programming. The diagnostic experience provides an excellent opportunity for professionals to address the concerns of parents given the child's developmental disabilities. Parents of special-needs children often identify skills in the preschool child that professionals do not recognize or credit. This is the time when parents and professionals can begin to either move together in their perceptions and viewpoints or move apart. Professionals need to explain the types of assessment tools utilized and the terms and definitions of the various tools, as well as the significance of the testing results. One problem that parents describe involves the different perceptions and analyses performed by various professionals on the multi-disciplinary team (Bailey, 1987). This team often consists of a school psychologist, a speech/language pathologist, an occupational therapist or physical therapist, and a special education teacher (see Figure 2-3). Members of the team need to explain not only the results of their particular assessment but also how their results fit in with the total picture for the child. Parents need to understand the difference between delay, difference, and disorder in labeling a child. They need to understand the differences among the disabling conditions

Figure 2-3
Evaluation Process

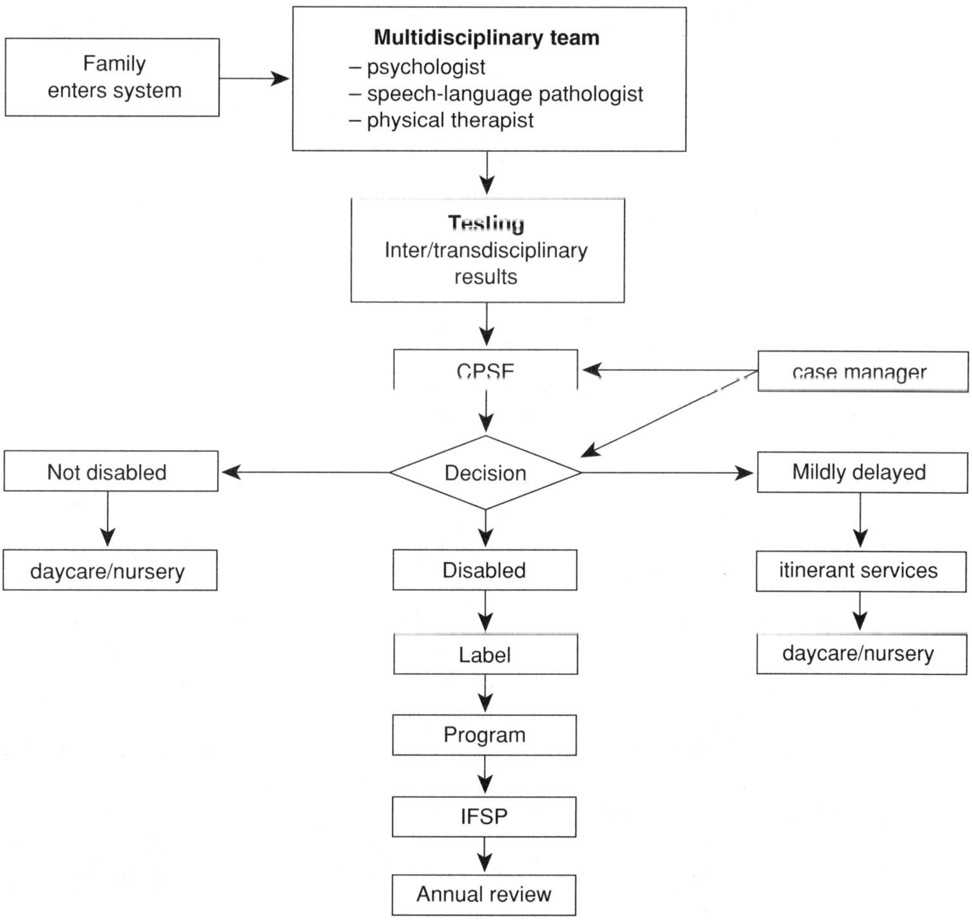

and how the multidisciplinary team arrived at the use of a specific disability label. The team should attempt to address the family's fears and concerns about having a child with developmental disabilities. This is not an exit conference with the team; it is the beginning of a lifelong process for the family. The team needs, therefore, to understand the role that *it* plays in setting the family correctly on its path. This is the time to answer such questions as "Will she ever talk?" "Will she ever read?" "Will she ever be normal?" It is important for the team to provide the family with realistic information so that parents have an opportunity to integrate the results of the evaluation process. Finally, it is important to stress the role of parents and the family in the educational development of the child and to assure parents that they play a very important role in the child's progress, growth, and development. Parents need to understand that there is a partnership, a long-term collaboration between parents and professionals—at home and at school (Donahue-Kilburg, 1992). All of this, of course, requires a certain amount of time with the family. The time set aside at the beginning of the process is indeed time well spent; it is here that the parent establishes an initial and very strong impression of the system.

PARENT-PROFESSIONAL RELATIONSHIPS

Changes in federal law as well as growing community consciousness have heightened awareness of persons with developmental disabilities. Consumer advocacy groups have also provided a mechanism for parents to change their role in the educational system (Yanok, 1986). The changing role of parents in education has been heightened by Public Law 99-457, which:

1. emphasizes a family-based program rather than a child-based program, and
2. stresses the significance of the parent functioning as an integral part in the process.

Perhaps there will be a healthy transaction when parents learn to assert their role in the educational system (Briggs, 1991). Just as parents have attitudes about professionals, professionals also have attitudes about parents. Figure 2-4 details the negative attitudes on both sides. If the parent-professional partnership is going to succeed, both must address and change their feelings.

Clearly, each side has concerns about the other. Parents are sensitive about not being respected for their efforts and their dreams. Professionals come from the perspective that parents need to follow through, carry over, and listen to the instructions. If parents are going to be partners in the process, then both sides need to develop a strong relationship in decision making. Clearly, there are many issues that influence the nature of the relationship between parents

Figure 2-4
Parental and Professional Attitudes

Parental Attitudes	Professional Attitudes
1. "There are no two professionals who agree."	1. "Just as the child is disabled, the parent is disabled."
2. "Each therapist has a specific ax to grind."	2. "The parent is responsible for the disabled child's problems."
3. "Professionals only focus on my child's deficits and disabilities—my child never has any strengths."	3. "The parent does not work hard enough and is not committed to change."
4. "Professionals do not understand that I have to do other things in my life than toilet-train my child six times a day. I have other children, a husband, a household."	4. "The parent is inconsistent and lazy."
5. "Professionals do not understand that I am a single parent and it is my child who is disabled. I am not disabled."	5. "The parent does not spend enough time with the disabled child."
6. "I find that professionals are impatient and intolerant; they see things only from their own vantage point."	6. "Parents expect miracles."
7. "I find that professionals do not understand that there is a long-term issue with a disabled child. They are too narrow in their focus and too short-term in their viewpoint."	7. "Parents are never satisfied. The only thing they want is a normal child."
	8. "Parents cannot accept the disabled child as he is."

and professionals. The primary attitudes that must be changed if a partnership is to be achieved are

- mutual respect
- mutual competence
- mutual commitment

Mutual Respect

Parents proceed through a grief process that is constant, long-term, and episodic (see Figure 2-5). Professionals must learn to understand what the life cycle is for parents of a disabled child. Dreams are broken with the realization that the child is not normal. Each parent must learn to accept the child and the fact that the developmental process for the whole family will be significantly

Figure 2-5
Parental Reaction

. . . Guilt (could it have been avoided?); sadness (would he be labeled unjustly?)

. . . I felt sad and somewhat depressed that my son was not "normal." What would he be like as an adult?

. . . We have three sons with learning disabilities. Our oldest is now seventeen years old and was nonfunctioning in his kindergarten class. We were devastated. I thought I had done something wrong. I felt I had a perfect child. My self-esteem as a mother was gone.

. . . I was depressed and scared. How would I be able to manage? How would by husband handle his son's deficit? I was afraid my husband would blame me or leave.

. . . Somewhat saddened. As a single parent trying to raise two young children without a father present, I felt there were now two strikes against my son. Luckily, my son was blessed with a sweet and loving demeanor and his happy natured personality makes things easier.

. . . We were upset; also confused about what the problem (and its cause) actually was, and concerned about when and if our son would be "cured."

. . . After the devastation, then the "why me." I realized how much he needed me, and I didn't have time to feel sorry for myself any more. Our oldest daughter, Kristen, seven at the time, asked "Why does my brother have to be so sick, why do we have a sick baby?" And before I could answer, she answered herself. "I know why, because God knows we will love him no matter what." It was those few words that changed my outlook. We weren't burdened, we were chosen. Every parent has to find a way of rationalizing the birth of a preschool child with disabilities.

different. In addition, the presence of a disabled child in a family is extremely stressful; many expectations about life, college, marriage, grandchildren, and so forth will be altered. There is a very high incidence of divorce in families with disabled children. Part of the learning process for parents must involve professional sensitivity to these issues and attention to teaching parents how to accept, how to proceed, how to cope. Parents have a great deal to contribute about the child's growth and learning. They can provide observations and experiences that are important to educational decision making. They should be involved as contributors to the child's and the educational team's process. Professionals must learn about the parental process and accept the parents for their attitudes and insights. With acceptance comes mutual respect on both sides (Healy, Keesee, & Smith, 1989).

Mutual Competence

Public Law 99-457 mandates the development of an IFSP* with the focus clearly on family-centered goals and issues (Donahue-Kilburg, 1992). The child must be viewed in the framework of home, siblings, parent or parents, and the economic variables in the environment. Parents are going to be influenced by

*An IFSP is an individualized service plan or program generated by the childcare committee. It outlines services and goals to meet the family's dynamic needs along with those of the child.

their interactions with professionals. Parents of disabled children have very different needs from those of parents of nondisabled children. In fact, the process and system that may work to educate nondisabled children may not work with children with developmental disabilities. Parents of disabled children must be trained, must be educated, must be empowered to function in a facilitative role. Parents are often passive, frightened, and uninvolved because they do not have enough knowledge to question the system or to question professionals in the system. Competency skills for parents must be knowledge-based. Parents must be systematically trained to function as educators, parents, and advocates for their children (Fitzgerald & Karnes, 1987).

Parents do not come equipped with the knowledge of effective parenting skills. Parents of nondisabled children learn through the trials and tribulations of normal dyactic-developmental interactions. They do not have the benefit of feedback from a normally developing child. The disabled child is often behaviorally impaired, unresponsive, and nonverbal. Professionals go to school for years to learn about the management of these issues. Parents of disabled children unfortunately must learn to fend for themselves (Healy, 1983). Early intervention programs must develop parent-education curricula that address the changing role of the parent. When the parent is educated, the nature of the interaction between parent and professional changes dramatically and dynamically; each contributes as an independent and interdependent member.

Mutual Commitment

With knowledge comes empowerment and effective functioning—independent functioning (Slentz, Walker, & Bricker, 1989). Parents can function as independent facilitators but they must be trained to do so. The attitude that must be changed by professionals involves the lazy parent—the one who wants to drop the child off to be "fixed." The educational system, particularly for children from five to twenty-one, has fostered dependence and passivity in parents because the focus has been on the child and on control by professionals. Many parents who proceed through a CSE* process for a school-age child describe the horrors of professional dominance at a meeting that does not permit parents even a voting right. It is clear at a CSE meeting that parents may "participate" but they may not vote. It is clear who makes the decision at a CSE meeting—the professionals and not the parents (Yanok & Derubertis, 1989).

If education is going to take parents seriously, and if professionals truly want parents to function as participants, they must from the very beginning accept the fact that parents are committed to the process of child change, growth, and development. The proviso here, however, is that when parents are empowered they become an independent force to be reckoned with. The parent cannot be a "patsy" for professional agreement and ease; he or she is entitled to

*A CSE, or committee on special education, is a mandated multidisciplinary school-based team that decides on educational placement for children who are disabled.

an opinion and a viewpoint, and ultimately is entitled to disagree with the professional (Healy, Keesee, & Smith, 1989). PL 99-457 provides an extraordinary opportunity for parents and professionals involved with early intervention to change their interaction and the decision-making process. For a preschool child, the law describes a different relationship between the CPSE (Committee on Preschool Special Education) and the parent. Clearly parental independence will affect the nature and the process of decision making for the team; here the parent is a committed part of the team.

Parents and Decision Making

If we want parents to contribute to the educational process, professionals must allow them to function as decision makers. This means parents contribute collaboratively to a team effort (Dunst, Trivette, & Deal, 1988). Decision making must evolve from the contributions of all members of the team. Public Law 99-457 contributes to the changing role of parents, since the emphasis is on collaborative decision making. Early intervention programs must train their professionals to share decisions with parents. Parents and professionals must learn *how* to make mutual decisions so that the individual expertise of each member contributes to the educational growth of the child (Winton, 1988). It is difficult for professionals to relinquish control of educational decision making, but the benefits for the child and for the educational system are tremendous (Donahue-Kilburg, 1992). Parents represent an untapped natural resource for

Figure 2-6
Parents' Thoughts on the Decision-Making Process

. . . In the decision making for my preschool language disordered child. As a parent to have my input accepted and incorporated.

. . . Open communication between parent and teacher. It's important to know what is being taught in school so that it can be reinforced at home.

. . . Involving yourself with the school—going to meetings, working with the teachers, and giving input if necessary.

. . . To advocate and become involved in SEPTAs and political process to guarantee special education and Boces and private schools are still available for a severely disabled child.

. . . Language is an integral part of the learning process. While Steven is obtaining these skills at school, I am reinforcing them at home.

. . . I don't believe the word *disabled* should make a difference in the role a parent plays in supporting the education of a child. Parents take on an unwritten obligation when they become a parent. Education is a major part.

. . . I can learn as a parent. I wanted to contribute to educational decisions. I know what is best for my child.

. . . I want to be respected and to be accepted as an important member of the committee and as a contributor to my child's education.

education. They can accomplish at home what the professional cannot, and without a doubt they are entitled to be recognized as equal partners. Learning to make decisions collaboratively will not be easy for parents or professionals. Negotiating is complex but worthwhile for all. The ability of the parents to contribute to the decision-making process is based on their knowledge and expertise (see Figure 2-6). This is the real challenge for education—transforming the role of the parent (Vincent, 1984).

SUMMARY

This chapter has discussed the changing role of the family in education and the fact that education as a whole is going through many changes. The issues faced by parents of disabled children are real issues faced by *all* parents whose children attend school. The problems in the American family are very similar to problems faced by teachers in schools. It is critical to understand that today's student, who will be the teacher of tomorrow, must face these changes and must understand the history as well as the basis for parent empowerment and child advocacy. Let us look forward and view these changes as a positive movement: the realignment of parent and professional. Let us look forward to a time when parents and professionals can share in the decision-making process, since the ultimate investment is the product of both—the child.

A FEW WORDS FROM TOYA DAVIS

As a parent of a disabled child I feel I have learned a great deal about the educational process and about empowerment in the process. I feel that I have been very fortunate since the program that my Jonathan attended took the issue of parent training and advocacy seriously. The school viewed the parent as the primary facilitator in a child's life and, as a result, they provided parent-education programs and peer support groups for mothers and fathers. I attended the parent-training classes with many other parents; classes were scheduled during the day and the evening so that parents with different work schedules could be accommodated.

The parent-education class was taught by Dr. Tiegerman and her professional staff. There was a structured curriculum that was similar to Dr. Tiegerman's graduate courses at the university in language development and language disorders. The academic lectures were combined with classroom observations, since the school had a closed-circuit video system and a television camera in every classroom. I could learn about pragmatic communicative functions in the parent-training class and then observe how communication behaviors were facilitated in Jonathan's class. There were reading assignments, lectures, and examinations. I learned about what it means to be language disordered as a child. I learned how to teach Jonathan at home and in contexts outside of school. I became one of Jonathan's teachers; I could actively participate in his growth and development. I felt invigorated, mobilized, and empowered by my new responsibility and role. Perhaps one of the greatest compliments that I ever received occurred after a conversation with the chairperson of my district's CSE. He asked me if I were a speech/language pathologist. I had learned to be a teacher and an advocate for Jonathan, skills that I could take with me as Jonathan progressed through his educational career. I knew that I could and would always be there for him as an active contributor. I feel that I have learned enough about the educational system and my son's learning difficulties that I can function as an effective advocate.

The educational system with all of its rules, regulations, and laws is very complicated. When parents enter the system they are initially overwhelmed by the fact that their child is disabled. The fact that the system is so complicated is an additional burden for families entering the process. I believe that parents must be incorporated into the child's education. I believe that all parents should be trained and educated whether the child is in special education, regular education, or gifted programming. I have learned that, as Jonathan's advocate, I can only function effectively if I know about my child and his learning problems. I can only contribute to his education if I know about educational procedures and techniques. I can only be a decision maker if I have enough knowledge to make a decision. I feel that educational programs and schools around the country should develop education classes for parents.

REFERENCES

Bailey, D. B., & Simeonsson, R. J. (1988). *Family assessment in early intervention.* New York: Merrill/Macmillan.

Bailey, D. (1987). Collaborative goal-setting with families: Resolving differences in values and priorities for services. *Topics in Early Childhood Special Education, 7,* 59–71.

Bailey, D. (1991). Issues and perspectives on family assessment. *Infants and Young Children, 4,* 26–34.

Barona, A., & Garcia, E. (Eds.) (1990). *Children at risk: Poverty, minority status, and other issues in educational equity.* Washington, DC: National Association of School Psychologists.

Brady, E. H. (1977). Home-school relations and continuity. *Theory into Practice, 16,* 41-46.

Briggs, M. (1991). Team development: Decision-making for early intervention. *Infant-Toddler Intervention: The Transdisciplinary Journal, 1,* 1–9.

Brinckerhoff, J. L., & Vincent, L. J. (1986). Increasing parental decision-making at the individualized educational program meeting. *Journal of the Division for Early Childhood, 11,* 46–58.

Bronfenbrenner, U. (1977). Toward an experimental ecology of human development. *American Psychologist, 32,* 513–531.

Cross, T. (1977). Mothers' speech adjustments: The contribution of selected child listener variables. In C. Snow & C. Ferguson (Eds.), *Talking to children.* London: Cambridge University Press.

Donahue-Kilburg, Gail. (1992). *Family-centered early intervention for communication disorders: Prevention and treatment.* Gaithersburg, MD: Aspen Publishing.

Dunst, C. J. (1985). Rethinking early intervention. *Analysis and Intervention in Developmental Disabilities, 5,* 165–201.

Dunst, C., Trivette, C., & Deal, A. (1988). Enabling and empowering families: Principles and guidelines for practice. Cambridge, MA: Brookline Books.

Edmonds, R. (1983). Quoted in U. Neisser (Ed.), *The school achievement of minority children: New perspectives* (pp. 1-17). Hillsdale, NJ: Erlbaum.

Edwards, P. A. (1987). Working with families from diverse backgrounds. In D. S. Strickland & E. J. Cooper (Eds.), *Educating black children: America's challenge* (pp. 92–104). Washington, DC: Howard University, Bureau of Educational Research, School of Education.

Edwards, P. (1990). Strategies and techniques for establishing home-school partnerships with minority parents. In A. Barona & E. Garcia (Eds.), *Children at risk: Poverty, minority status, and other issues in educational equity.* Washington, DC: National Association of School Psychologists.

Fitzgerald, M. T., & Karnes, D. E. (June 1987). A parent-implemented language model for at risk and developmentally delayed preschool children. *Topics in Language Disorders.*

Fuchs, D., Fuchs, L. S., Power, M. H., & Dailey, A. M. (1985). Bias in the assessment of handicapped children. *American Educational Research Journal, 22,* 185–198.

Healy, A. (1983). *The needs of children with disabilities: A comprehensive view.* Iowa City: University of Iowa Press.

Healy, A., Keesee, P., & Smith, B. (1989). Early services for children with special needs: Transactions for family support. Iowa City: University Hospital School.

Kaiser, A., & Blair, G. (1987). Mother-child transactions in families with normal and handicapped children. *Uppsala Journal of Medical Science, 44,* 204–207.

Krauss, M. W. (1990). New precedent in family policy: Individualized family service plan. *Exceptional Children, 56,* 388–395.

Lynch-Fraser, D., & Tiegerman, E. (1987). *Babysignals.* New York: Walker Publishing Company.

McDade, H., & Varnedoe, D. R. (1987). Training parents to be language facilitators. *Topics in Language Disorders, 7,* 19–30.

McDade, H. L., & Varnedoe, D. R. (June 1987). A parent-implemented language model for at-risk and developmentally delayed preschool children. *Topics in Language Disorders.*

Miranda, A. H., & Santos de Barona, M. (1990). A model for interventions with low achieving minority students. In A. Barona & E. Garcia (Eds.), *Children at risk* (pp. 119–133). Washington, DC: National Association of School Psychologists.

National Center for Family-Centered Care (1990). *What is family-centered care?* (Brochure). Washington, DC: Association for the Care of Children's Health.

National Commission on Excellence in Education (1983). *A nation at risk: The imperative for educational reform.* Washington, DC: U.S. Department of Education.

Neisser, U. (1986). New answers to an old question. In U. Neisser (Ed.), *The school achievement of minority children: New perspectives* (pp. 1–17). Hillsdale, NJ: Erlbaum.

Public Law 99-457. (1986). Education of the handicapped act amendments of 1986, Title I, Handicapped infants and toddlers. Washington, DC: House Congressional Record.

Sameroff, A. J., & Chandler, M. J. (1975). Reproductive risk and the continuum of caretaking causality. In F. D. Horowitz, M. Hetherington, S. Scarr-Salapatek, & G. Siegel (Eds.), *Review of child development research* (Vol. 4, pp. 187–244). Chicago: University of Chicago Press.

Sexton, D., Miller, J. H., & Rotatori, A. F. (1985). Determinants of professional-parental agreement for the developmental status of young handicapped children. *Journal of Psychoeducational Assessment, 4,* 377–390.

Slentz, K., Walker, B., & Bricker, D. (1989). Supporting parent involvement in early intervention: A role-taking model. In G. Singer and L. Irvin (Eds.), *Support for caregiving families enabling positive adaptation to disability* (pp. 207–219). Baltimore, MD: Paul H. Brookes.

Tiegerman, E., & Siperstein, M. (September 1984). Individual patterns of interaction in the mother-child dyad: Implications for parent intervention. *Topics in Language Disorders.*

Vincent, E. (1984). Family relationship. In *Equals in this partnership: Parents of disabled and at-risk infants and toddlers speak to professionals.* Washington, DC: National Center for Clinical Infant Programs.

Vohs, J. (1989). Recommendations for working with families and children with special needs from diverse cultures and organizational resources for understanding families from diverse cultures. In B. Hanft (Ed.), *Family-centered care—an early intervention resource manual* (pp. 67, 69–74). Rockville, MD: The American Occupational Therapy Association.

Winton, P. (1988). Effective communication between parents and professionals. In D. Bailey and R. Simeonsson (Eds.), *Family assessment in early intervention* (pp. 207–228). New York: Merrill/Macmillan.

Yanok, J. (1986). Free appropriate public education for handicapped children: Congressional intent and judicial interpretation. *Remedial and Special Education, 7,* 49–53.

Yanok, J., & Derubertis, D. (1989). Comparative study of parental participation in regular and special education programs. *Exceptional Children,* 195–199.

Yell, M., & Espin, C. (1990). The handicapped children's protection act of 1986: Time to pay the piper? *Exceptional Children, 56,* 396–407.

Yoshida, R. K., Fenton, K. S., Kaufman, M. J., & Maxwell, J. P. (1978). Parental involvement in special education pupil planning process: The school's perspective. *Exceptional Children, 44,* 531–534.

CHAPTER

3

EDUCATION LAWS AND PROCEDURES

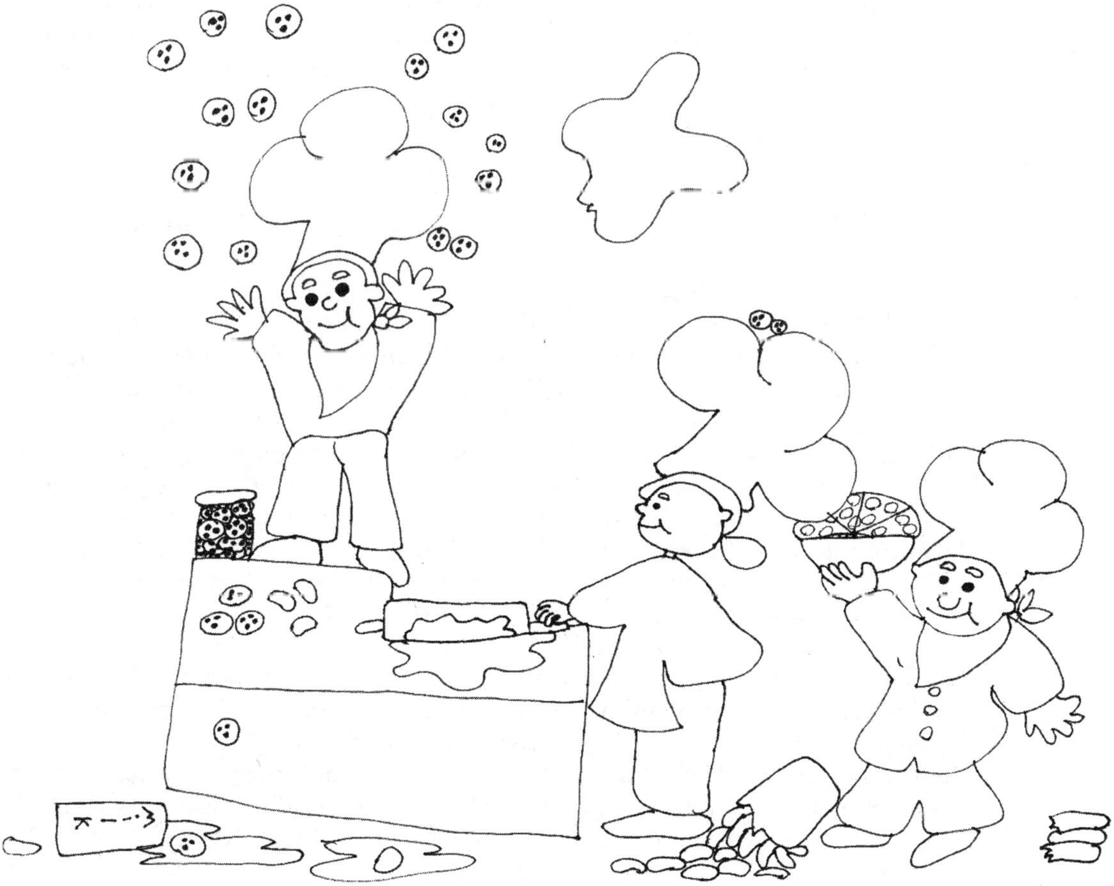

The purpose of this chapter is to consider some of the social, legal, and educational issues that influence early intervention services.

LANDMARK LEGISLATION FOR THE DISABLED

Education has been faced with dynamic legal requirements that ultimately have resulted in programmatic changes at all levels for disabled and nondisabled children. **Public Law 94-142,** the Education for All Handicapped Children Act of 1975, and **Public Law 93-112,** the Rehabilitation Act of 1973, Section 504, are considered to be the declaration of civil rights for all disabled children and adults (Sarason, 1982). Originally, Section 504 defined a disabled individual only in regard to employment; that is, disabled persons were entitled to employment opportunities and discrimination because of disabling conditions was illegal. This definition was expanded, however, in 1974, when it was amended under the Rehabilitation Act Amendments of 1974 **(Public Law 93-516)**. The definition under this amendment included education, meaning that disabled persons were entitled to educational opportunities, and discrimination based on disabling conditions was now illegal and a violation of a person's civil rights.

Education for All Handicapped Children Act

The laws clearly and unambiguously stated that disabled individuals have equal rights to education and employment. No longer can disabled children be excluded from educational opportunities because of a disabling condition. The Education for All Handicapped Children Act **(EAHCA)** of 1975 was enacted to assist states in providing disabled children with a free and appropriate public education **(F.A.P.E.)**. The EAHCA establishes minimum requirements that must be complied with in order for states to be eligible to receive financial assistance. Each state must have "in effect a policy that assures all disabled children the right to free appropriate public education" (20 U.S.C. Section 1412 [1]), "and must develop a plan which details the policies and procedures which ensure the provider of that right" (Section 1412 [2]).

Each state must also establish procedural safeguards (Section 1412 [5]) in order to ensure that local educational agencies in that state will create the individualized educational programs required by the Act (Section 1412 [4]). In essence, each state must formulate a plan for educating its disabled children, and that plan must be approved by the Secretary of Education before the state is entitled to federal funds. The EAHCA addressed a long-standing issue that affected the education of disabled children nationally. Specifically, local school districts often excluded children whose disabilities prevented them from participating in regular school programs.

Public Law 94-142 continues to be a primary force in maintaining the educational rights of disabled children throughout the United States. The law provides for four planning requirements:

1. The development of an Individualized Education Program (IEP);
2. The right to be educated in the Least Restrictive Environment (LRE);
3. The provision of appropriate related services dependent on educational and developmental needs; and
4. Parental involvement.

In 1991, Public Law 102-119 amended the directory language of Public Law 101-476 by substituting "Individuals with Disabilities Education Act" for "Education for the Handicapped Act." The change of EHCA to IDEA that all children with disabilities have available to them a free appropriate public education, with emphasis on special education and related services to meet their unique needs.

All of the rights and protections of Public Law 94-142 were extended to disabled preschoolers through the enactment of Public Law 99-457 in 1986. This new law provides an opportunity for the development of comprehensive service delivery systems specifically designed for disabled infants, toddlers, preschoolers, and their families. The passage of both bills should be viewed in the context of changing social policy and social attitudes. Great strides in early intervention programming occurred only after a great deal of personal and political struggle. This struggle resulted ultimately in passage of 94-142 and 99-457. The wonder and beauty of those laws are that they are a culmination of forty-five years of progress and enlightenment regarding how we deal with special-needs children and adults. It began in the post–WWII years when a burst of rehabilitative technology and medical intervention occurred. Multitudes of permanently disabled soldiers returned home and needed this new technology in order to reenter their society. In the early 1960s we had a president who had a severely disabled sister (Rosemary Kennedy). This child was much loved and respected by her family and we learned through their model about the integrity of the disabled person.

The Rehabilitation Act of 1974

In the Civil Rights movement of the latter 1960s, we learned about the integrity and rights of all persons regardless of color or religion. In 1973 the civil rights of all disabled individuals were clarified in Section 504 of the Rehabilitation Act, Public Law 93-112. In its original version this law applied only to discrimination in the workplace. However, in 1974, it was amended to forbid

Figure 3-1
Foundations for Educational Legislation

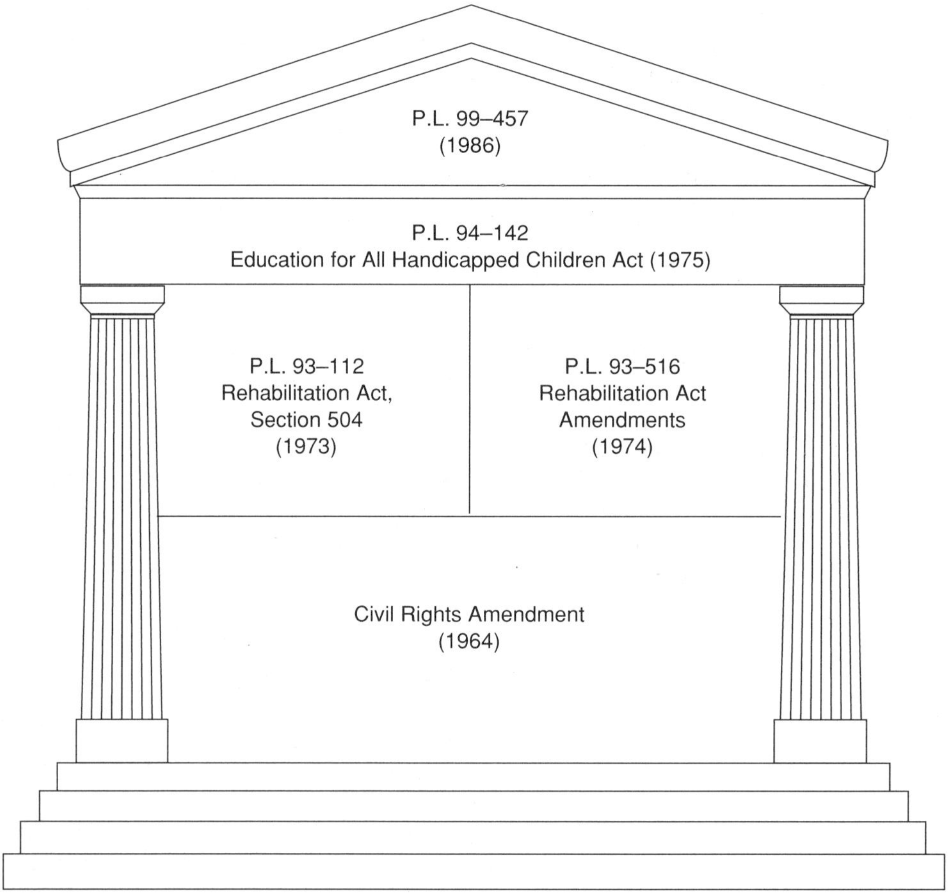

discrimination of the disabled not only in the workplace, but in all educational settings as well. All of these laws have ensured increased services for disabled persons. Figure 3-1 depicts how these laws built a solid structure of educational guaranties and entitlements for disabled persons in the United States. These increased services, however, must be contrasted on an ongoing basis with changes in the economic climate and resources (White, 1986).

The passage of socially based legislation is usually a function of aggressive advocacy by special interest groups of parents, families, and professionals. Healy, Keesee, and Smith (1989) note that often legislative policy is at odds with social demands—"the concrete measure of policy is financial" (p. 87). During periods of crisis, the most enlightened of policies that initially created programs are just not funded. The ultimate impact on children and families is the same as not having the policy at all; services are eliminated.

Several decades ago disabled people were institutionalized. Today, social attitudes have changed so dramatically that institutionalization is the final item on a long list of educational and placement alternatives. Research has revealed that institutionalization can result in the lowering of cognitive abilities, and, because the most likely areas to be affected are verbal abilities and abstract thinking (Balla, 1976; Butterfield, 1967; Zigler, 1973), we must prevent this from happening. Consequently, educational research and programming have provided support for two basic principles:

1. Disabled individuals can be educated and trained to function in society.
2. The earlier the intervention process begins, the more efficacious the results.

In describing the results of almost two decades of programming since the passage of Public Law 94-142, it is important to note that economic problems have resulted in restrictions in eligibility criteria. This means that, nationally, at-risk and mildly disabled children are denied services because they are not "disabled enough," that is, severely disabled. Healy and colleagues (1989) note that the public is very likely to cut first preventive and maintenance care and health programs that reach children and the poor. This is unfortunate, since the developmental outcome of high-risk infants often includes increased susceptibility to physical and developmental deficits such as educational difficulties, deficient parent-infant bonding, behavioral abnormalities, abuse, and neglect (Rosetti, 1986).

BASES FOR EARLY INTERVENTION

Several researchers have investigated how changing the early environment and structuring the developmental experiences for children might influence their later development. Such studies provide insights into the role of early intervention with the disabled as well as the importance of such experiences for nondisabled children in day care and preschool programs (Meisels, 1985). One important question that researchers have attempted to answer relates to whether early facilitation has a substantial influence on long-term developmental and educational issues. Many investigations have demonstrated that early intervention does have long-term influence on children's functioning (Bloom, 1964; Hunt, 1961; Kirk, 1958; Skeels, 1966). It has been noted that these studies are difficult to compare given methodological differences. The results, however, support the concept that early stimulation can increase development and that environmental difficulties can negatively impact on children's growth and education.

The need for documentation for early intervention programming has generated a great deal of research. Palmer (1977) noted that preschool children with early facilitative experiences had significantly higher IQs and achievement scores than children without such experiences. Perhaps one of the best-known studies has been the Ypsilanti Perry Preschool Project. This long-term investigation indicated that mildly disabled and disadvantaged high-risk children who were placed in preschool programs showed developmental and educational gains that continued into the public school years. In fact, 39 percent of the children who did not attend preschool were later placed in special education classes as compared to only 19 percent of those who attended preschool. Perhaps most striking, given the demands of economic constraints, were the educational costs involved. There were significant cost savings in educating a special-needs child earlier, since fewer years of special education resulted afterwards. The principle is simple: If society does not identify and educate early, the problem becomes more severe later. Such results support the position that society cannot afford to wait to remediate (see Figure 3-2) (Marozas & May, 1988).

While the data on the efficacy of early intervention programs have been available for several decades, the lack of funding for children's programming obviously becomes a function of economic factors rather than program effectiveness (Marozas & May, 1988). The sentiment concerning disabled and nondisabled children often dwindles along with funding during periods of financial austerity. The realities of children's programming should not be based on the financial climate of American society, since this presents a rather limited and short-term perspective on social issues. In the business arena we have learned from other countries that business success is best measured not by an immediate huge return, but by a slow, steady increase in profit and market. It takes a long-term commitment with a focus on quality in order to be successful. So it is in the area of education and social policy. America needs to develop a national policy on children and thereby make a long-term commitment to its most precious resource—the future of its children.

Anastasiow (1986) argued that the efficacy of early intervention focuses on the wrong issue. Efficacy becomes the central issue when there is not a social and moral commitment to children. American society must view education as a lifelong process that enriches families as well as our cultural heritage. A short-term perspective shortchanges our contribution as a society to world affairs. Unfortunately, programs for children are not usually protected from political and social influences. One pressing problem appears to be the lack of a comprehensive national policy for children in the United States. Other countries, such as Sweden and Israel, have made a national commitment to children; children are viewed as a future investment and resource. Because of the absence of such a comprehensive child policy, laws have been passed as a result of active lobbying, and parents and professionals have had to form alliances to raise the consciousness level of policy makers in government (Dublinske, 1989). Change does not come easily. It should be remembered that the Education for All Handicapped Children Act (EAHCA) was passed only after many years of political activism

Figure 3-2
What Is the Benefit of Early Intervention to Society?

. . . Early intervention is everything. When a person is exposed to things early on, things come easier.

. . . I don't know *yet*. I can only imagine that it will enable my son to be a productive member. As in any "diagnosis and treatment" the earlier something is dealt with, the better the results.

. . . The earlier the intervention, the less emotional loss of self-esteem; the better chance of helping the child to cope with his or her disabling condition. The better the chance to help the child to develop strategies to cope with the disability.

. . . The younger the child is, the easier it is for the child to learn. The child doesn't have an existing way of doing things. The older the child is, the more problems that have to be corrected and the harder it is to change a predetermined attitude. As a result, more intervention is needed, resulting in more loss to society.

. . . Early intervention might curtail the need for intensive therapy in grade school and high school.

. . . The children will lead normal lives in the public schools, by not being in "special class" for the school years.

. . . It will facilitate the child's entry into mainstream education, thus preventing the need for resource room, special education, and other expensive programs over a longer period of time.

. . . Makes children ready to accept education (gives them the basic tools to learn) without which there is no foundation and wastes time and money in the school system.

. . . In my work as a volunteer parent member I have seen what early intervention has done to improve the potential for some students. If they haven't received help by three or four their self-esteem suffers and adults with low self-esteem emerge from our schools as failures.

. . . There is a greater chance of these children going on to regular classes and costing society less in special education later. The longer you wait the more work the child will need.

. . . Early intervention maximizes the opportunity to produce a self-sufficient adult. It also alleviates the costs of much adult education and supportive services.

. . . An early treatment leads to an early "cure" or early adaptation to the disabling condition. Less psychological damage and better self-esteem is a result of helping children and their families to understand what is happening to them and how to deal with it.

. . . The past two years Steven has been in special programs, I have seen him come a long way. When he first went to preschool he couldn't speak a word; he would struggle to get a sound out. His eyes would fill with tears as the frustration would set in. These children need the special attention to come into their own. I know Steven will eventually be in a mainstream environment and develop to his full potential. I'm certain Steven will be able to be whatever he wants to be in life.

(see Figure 3-3). Let us then consider the education laws and procedures described below. They are often complex and confusing and complicated by social activism and the pressures of legislative decision making. With this all in mind, we begin our special education ABCs.

EDUCATION PROCEDURES

Congress was not explicitly clear in the EAHCA as to what exactly constitutes an "appropriate" education, and often parents and school districts do not agree on what is "appropriate" to meet the educational needs of a particular disabled child

Figure 3-3
Timeline of Events Leading to IDEA

1945	Post–WW II Period
1964	Civil Rights Amendment
1973	PL 93-112, Rehab Act, Section 504
1974	PL 93-516, Rehab Act Amendments
1975	PL 94-142, Education for ALL Handicapped Children Act
1986	PL 99-457
1990	ADA, Americans with Disabilities Act
1991	Implementation of Infant based services
	IDEA Individuals with Disabilities Education Act

(Yanok, 1986). The U.S. Supreme Court case of **Board of Education v. Rowley** established a standard for evaluating the appropriateness of a disabled child's education; specifically, that the child's program must allow him or her to receive educational benefits. The Rowley case involves an eight-year-old deaf child whose parents claimed that she was entitled to have a sign language interpreter in her classroom to enable her to have the same educational opportunity as her classmates. The Supreme Court held that EAHCA is satisfied when a school provides personalized instruction within sufficient support services to permit the disabled child to benefit educationally from that instruction. The court stated that the EAHCA was not meant to guarantee a disabled child a certain level of education but merely to open the door of education to disabled children by means of special education services. In the case of Amy Rowley, it was determined that she was receiving educational programming that enabled her to achieve passing grades and advance to the next grade. Under EAHCA a school is not required to maximize the potential of a disabled child, nor is it required to provide equal educational opportunity commensurate with the opportunity provided to nondisabled children. EAHCA provides only for baseline requirements; interestingly, some states have educational standards that surpass the federal standards (Data Research, 1988). *Appropriate,* then, is an ambiguous term that clearly results in programming differences from school district to school district and from state to state. Consequently, a grave responsibility rests on the **Committee on Preschool Special Education (CPSE)** and the **Committee on Special Education (CSE)** to provide the disabled child with educational programming that is individualized to meet the needs of the child. When parents of disabled children are not satisfied with the educational plan that the committee generates, parents and committees need to negotiate to find a mutually agreeable plan. If they are unable to do so, parents have the option of due process, which will be explained later in this chapter (Mayer, 1982).

Least Restrictive Environment

The most difficult and perhaps the most controversial issue in the placement of disabled children involves the definition of *least restrictive environment* (LRE). To make matters even more complicated, the term **least restrictive environment** is often confused with **mainstreaming** and **regular education initiative (REI).** In order to clarify some of the issues, let us begin with the term *mainstreaming* and its definition.

Mainstreaming reflects a long-term developmental process in the educational life of the disabled child. With the continuum of services, the mainstreaming process means the gradual transition of the disabled child from the more **restrictive (special) placement** to the regular (nondisabled) classroom. As the child progresses along the placement continuum, he becomes ready for the challenges of regular education and socialization with nondisabled peers. There is an attempt by school districts to "integrate" children with disabilities into regular school, classes, and programs. Although mainstreaming is not mandated by specific state statute, both federal regulations and commissioners' regulations (in various states) require that "to the maximum extent appropriate" special education be provided in the least restrictive environment (Hageny, 1986). Most recently **inclusion programming,** a new concept regarding integration of disabled and nondisabled youngsters in the educational setting, has arisen. It differs from mainstreaming in regard to academic expectations. Mainstreaming implies that the disabled child is ready to manage the same academic curriculum as the nondisabled students in the classroom through the facilitation of appropriate support services. Inclusion programming implies that a disabled child can be integrated with nondisabled children without the expectation of his or her managing the same academic curriculum as nondisabled students. Rather, an individualized set of academic goals will be generated for the disabled child and these goals will be met in the regular education classroom.

To date, inclusion programming has not yet taken a strong hold in the educational system. It remains to be seen what impact this full integration philosophy will have on special education in the next few years. Inclusion purists have a slogan: "Inclusion for all disabled children. What part of *all* don't you understand?"

The EAHCA requires that states provide procedures to ensure that disabled children are educated "to the maximum extent appropriate" with nondisabled children in regular classes. Difficulties in the learning process are to be addressed by the provision of special aides and support services rather than by separate schooling for the disabled. Courts prefer to uphold a "mainstreaming" decision where a child's educational needs can be met in the regular classroom (Data Research, 1988).

Federal law historically has described the least restrictive environment as the placement that meets the disabled child's individual needs. As part of the placement decision making, school districts should engage in a "rule out process," in which the district reviews whether or not there is an "appropriate" placement (a) in the district; (b) in a neighboring school district; (c) in public nondistrict programs; (d) in private schools; and, finally, (e) in residential facilities. In the process of decision making, the school district should not place a child in a program because it is public rather than private; the placement decision should be child-driven, not program-driven. However, in some states school districts make placement decisions not on the individual needs of the child but rather on the identification of a public program. This means that the individual needs of the disabled child are offset by public versus private program issues (Data Research, 1988).

LRE should be achievable anywhere, not only in public schools. It is quite clear that the primary issue for the disabled child must involve the prescriptive and the individual aspects that can facilitate learning. A disabled child is one who is not progressing through a normal developmental sequence and requires specialized instruction. "If my child could benefit from a regular class, he would have been able to learn without specialized instruction" (Toya Davis). A disabled child needs a learning environment that is tailored to him or her—individualized and prescriptive. An individualized and prescriptive educational setting can occur along a continuum of placements. Unfortunately, in most situations, LRE has often been interpreted to mean the regular educational classroom, regardless of individual needs.

Regular Education Initiative

The least restrictive environment issue becomes even more complicated with the introduction of the **Regular Education Initiative (REI)**. **Public Law 94-142** stipulates that all disabled children are guaranteed a free and appropriate public education **(F.A.P.E.)**. The intent of 94-142 was that a child identified as disabled would receive educational services along a placement continuum. The use of REI for disabled children proposes that the starting point must be the regular classroom. This would mean that the disabled child would have to fail in the regular classroom before he was removed for placement along the continuum. A document from New York State's Commissioner of Education states "separate school or removal from the regular education environment may occur only when the nature and severity of the disorder is such that education in regular classes cannot be satisfactorily achieved." The implication is quite clear; the child must first fail in the regular class in order to become a special education student.

What is not clear is how severely impaired the child must be in order to be removed. The intent of 94-142 was that the disabled child was to receive special education services because he was disabled—mildly, moderately, or severely. This initiative suggests a different intent. Here only the most severely disabled child can be referred for special education services. Here the child must fail first in the regular class before being considered for special education services. How much time will pass before the child will finally receive the services so desperately needed? Why must the disabled child fail first or at all? In addition, mildly and moderately disabled children will remain in the regular classroom because they are no longer disabled *enough* to receive special education services. The definition of *least restrictive environment* has changed over the years to reflect a number of political issues that had nothing to do with the individual needs of the disabled child—first mainstreaming and now REI.

Procedural Safeguards

States receiving federal funds under EAHCA must develop an Individualized Educational Program (IEP) for each disabled child. The IEP is generated by and annually reviewed by a Committee on Special Education (CSE). Each state utilizes a set of identification, evaluation, and operational procedures that make up the specific outline for state procedures being detailed in the Commissioner of Education's Regulations.

A school district Board of Education (BOE) is responsible for the education of all children in the school district; this includes disabled children. The Board of Education must identify and register all disabled children residing in the district and must also appoint a Committee on Special Education, establish policy for the provision of special education programs and services, and approve recommendations from the CSE.

The Committee on Special Education (CSE) is described as a multidisciplinary team with specific mandated responsibilities (see Figure 3-4).

a. The CSE is responsible for the evaluation of all children suspected of having a disabling condition.
b. The CSE is responsible for classifying and labeling the child who is in fact disabled.
c. The CSE must identify the appropriate educational program to meet the disabled child's individual needs.
d. The CSE must generate an individualized educational plan for the child and review that plan at least annually.

Figure 3-4
Committee on Special Education: Decision-Making Process

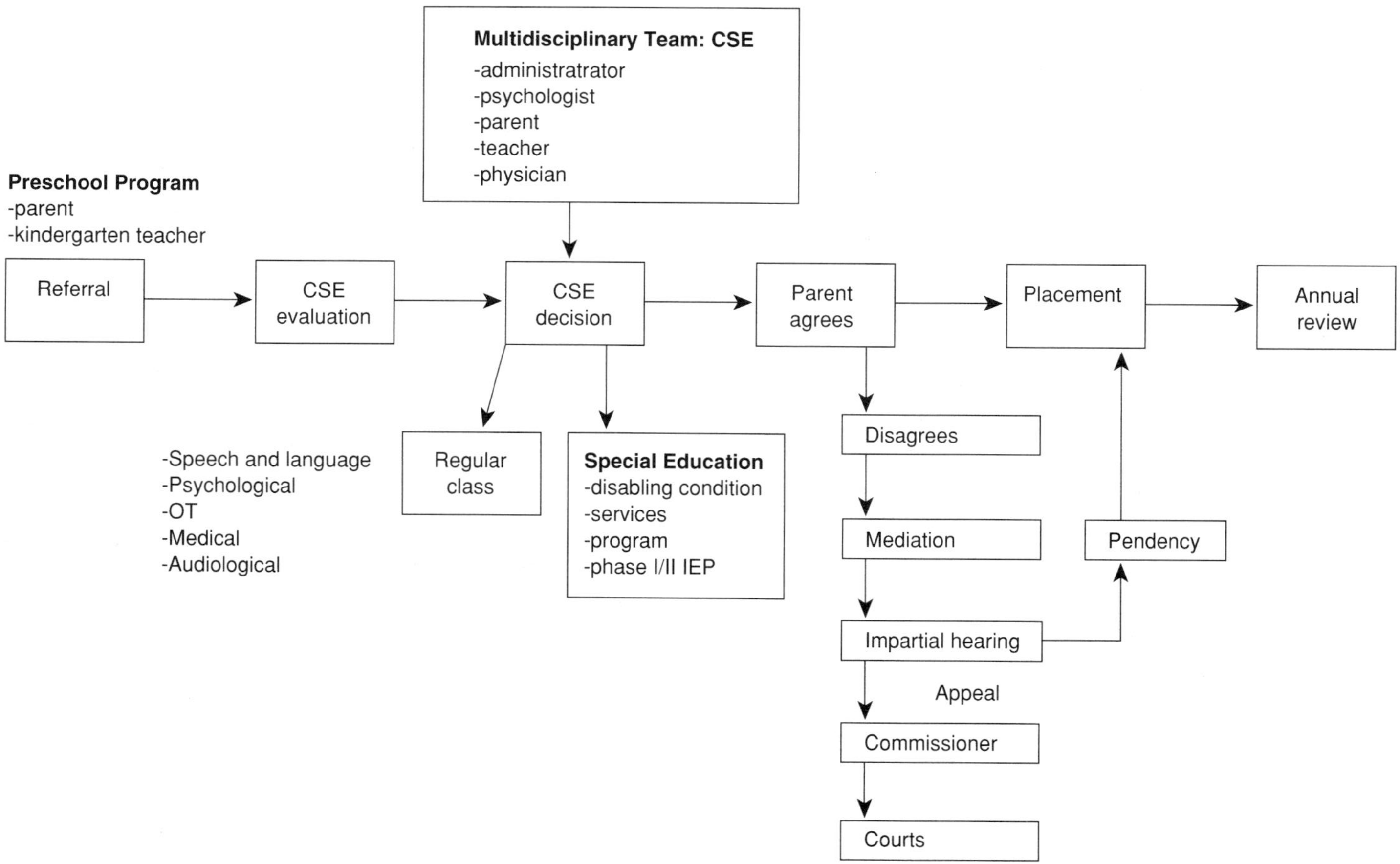

Figure 3-5
Is the CSE Process More Difficult than the CPSE Process?

. . . Our CSE process was NOT a difficult process. Prior to placement at SLCD, our committee asked that we look at our BOCES program, which we did. Then, using information learned in Parent Training, we explained why it was not an appropriate placement. Michael was then placed at SLCD. Continued placement for first and second grade was approved.

. . . The CSE process entails so much more than the CPSE process. More parental research is necessary at this point.

. . . Yes, because the school district incorporates itinerant services into the kindergarten program so their goal is to mainstream the child. In my situation, everyone was in agreement that my daughter was ready to be transitioned to kindergarten and received speech therapy three times a week.

. . . Yes, districts are trying to save money. If the parents don't know state regulations and aren't knowledgeable it can be a nightmare. It is very hard for me every time I go, unless I plan before. I do not achieve my goals for my three disabled children. If I don't advocate for them, no one will. Most parents either don't care or don't take time to find out about laws and regulations.

. . . Yes, because chairpeople are not as strict in placement during CPSE because there are so many preschools and all are private but in school-age public education they always want to keep the children away from "private school." It's like the curse word and the last possible thing they consider.

e. The CSE must determine the appropriate type and levels of services to meet the disabled child's educational needs.
f. The CSE has the responsibility to satisfy the least restrictive environment (LRE) requirements.

The Committee on Special Education should consider all evaluative information on the child in order to make an appropriate decision about his or her label, placement, and educational needs. The CSE is a very powerful committee with a "precious responsibility." The parent whose child is being evaluated by the CSE is often frightened and overwhelmed (see Figure 3-5). In fact, the role of the parent is rather ambiguously described in terms such as *participation* and *involvement*. The reality, however, is awesome; the committee votes, the parent does not. In fact, a CSE meeting can be held without a parent being present.

The Individualized Education Plan (IEP)

The IEP is a document that summarizes a child's current skills and abilities, establishes educational goals, and describes program components necessary to meet the child's needs. It is extremely important; it functions as the basis for instruction and is a contract between the parent and the school district that a specific program and services will be provided to the child.

The IEP, which is developed during a planning conference with parents, teachers, and specialists, functions as the teacher's ongoing instructional guide in order to meet the child's annual goals. Daily lessons and activities should relate specifically to short-term and long-term goals. For as long as the child remains in special education, the IEP is reviewed and modified on an annual basis.

Continuum of Services

Individualized Education Programs can be provided in various types of settings or placements. As stated previously, in the process of providing the disabled child with an individualized plan, the CSE must also take into consideration the issue of least restrictive environment and must identify the appropriate placement that meets the child's individual needs. The disabled child may be educated in any of the following placements depending on his or her educational needs:

- the regular education classroom;
- the regular education classroom with a consulting special education teacher;
- a special education classroom in the school district;
- a special education classroom in a neighboring school district;
- at home or in a hospital;
- nondistrict state-approved special schools;
- state-operated residential care facilities.

These educational programs provide a range of services along a placement continuum for disabled children. The options begin in the regular classroom. If the disabled child requires (a) more intensive individualized instruction and/or (b) rehabilitative services and/or (c) highly structured classroom instruction and/or (d) smaller class size and/or (e) modified curriculum programming, one of the other placement options would be considered as appropriate to meet the child's needs. Each of these placements is meant to meet the individual needs of the child. Although in the hierarchy of placements the regular education classroom is the least restrictive, any one of these settings can be the LRE for a special-needs child, depending on the needs of that child.

Personal Insights

The above sections have dealt with procedural issues, laws, and regulations, and some of the rationales underlying changes in the federal mandate. In sharing insights into the complexities of the educational process, it is hoped that some thought-provoking questions will be raised. Perhaps the most striking personal insight relates to the fact that the bureaucratic process for children and families in education is overwhelmingly complex. The laws and their ensuing state regulations are unfortunately ambiguous. Although the intent is to protect children with disabilities, the result is that each Committee on Preschool Special Education generates a recommendation for services and placement based on personal perceptions, individual biases, and community politics. Because of its ambiguities, the law must be interpreted in order to be applied in the real world. It is difficult for families to understand the ambiguities, the complexities, and the peculiarities that result in educational differences across various school districts. Whereas one school district may disapprove of placement, when a parent moves to another school district, placement is approved. As a result, there is a great deal of family movement from district to district based on which district will recommend and/or provide specific programs and services.

Another problem related to the complexity of the process is that unless parents are directly taught to understand the system, they remain ignorant of the process. There are no formal courses at universities or public schools that teach parents about the law, the bureaucratic system, and the due process procedures. Therefore, parents unfortunately are left to their own resources in finding out about how the system works. Often there is a network of parents that functions as a support group—parents helping parents to survive a complex system.

This is not just a system of rules, procedures, and laws; it is a system that must be interpreted and applied by people. Just as teachers and professionals must learn how to fairly represent the law, professionals must also understand how to separate political issues from child issues. Parents must learn to deal with the system as well as with their emotions. They must learn to channel their frustration and their anger. Public Law 94-142 in its spirit had a noble intent to equalize the opportunities and erase the discrimination for the disabled. Parents realize over time that there is a marked discrepancy between the spirit of the law and the letter of the law. Often the letter of the law is interpreted by school district professionals who have an agenda that does not necessarily coincide with the family's. The system finally only works when school issues, parent concerns, and child needs all overlap; this represents a remarkable struggle that can be achieved only when there is collaboration.

APPEAL PROCESS

Due Process

Due process describes the procedures used to ensure that the disabled child is provided a free and appropriate public education (F.A.P.E.). Due process consists of several assurances of **parental rights**:

1. The right to be fully informed and knowledgeable about the actions to be taken.

2. The right to participate in the determination of decisions through attendance at meetings.
3. The right to give or withhold consent.
4. The right to challenge school decisions.
5. The right to appeal the decision of an impartial hearing officer.

All of these due process rights are an integral part of the decision-making process. They should be viewed not only as rights, but as the responsibility of all parents of special-needs children. Federal law states that procedures must be established to ensure that parents of disabled children are informed and are given the opportunity to participate in decision making.

The CSE Meeting

Parents must be informed of their rights, as well as adequately notified of the CSE's proposed actions, purposes, and decisions concerning the child. Generally, when the parent appears before the committee, it is an intimidating and overwhelming experience. The CSE will discuss evaluation results, the child's level of functioning, and the child's educational needs, and ultimately decide on the appropriate placement for the child—clearly decision making by committee. The CSE is mandated to decide the educational future of the disabled child with or without the parent's agreement. It is shocking for many parents of disabled children to realize that when they appear before the CSE, they do not have a vote—only a voice. They can participate but they cannot ultimately vote. If the parent disagrees with the decision of the CSE, it is the parent's responsibility to challenge the committee. The parent has a basic right to challenge by requesting mediation or an impartial hearing.

The concept of questioning/challenging a CSE decision appears inherently adversarial and aggressive and one must remember that the special education child needs a responsible advocate. Parents as well as school districts need to recognize that the decision to exercise the due process right of an impartial hearing or mediation occurs after careful thinking and deliberation.

Special Education Mediation

In an attempt to assist committees on special education, boards of education, and responsible school officials to resolve disputes with parents without resorting to impartial hearings, which are quasi-legal proceedings, some states have piloted special education **mediation** as an interim procedure (see Figure 3-6). Many states are considering this process, which offsets the time and legal expenses related to an impartial hearing by providing a mechanism to clarify issues and concerns, areas of agreement and disagreement, and applicable

Figure 3-6
The Appeal Process

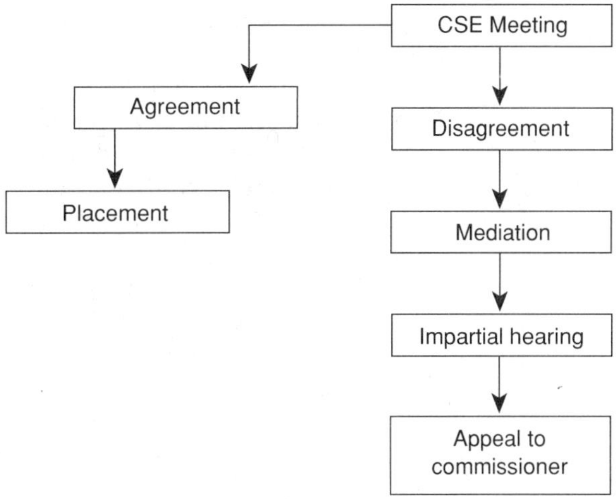

laws, regulations, and policies so that parents and school districts negotiate a resolution to the dispute rather than receiving a ruling from an "impartial" hearing officer. If the mediation process does not provide a workable solution, nothing prevents the parent from then requesting an impartial hearing. **Community Dispute Resolution Centers (CDRC)** have personnel who are well trained in issues relating to the rights and educational needs of children with disabling conditions and who provide an environment in which negotiation can be fostered and facilitated.

Impartial Hearing

An impartial hearing is a formal procedure used to resolve conflict between parents and school districts over the provision of special education. The impartial hearing has been established as a mechanism to hear both sides of the issues and resolve the dispute through a third party—the impartial hearing officer. This officer may not be an employee of the school district, but because he or she is chosen by and paid by the district, many parents question whether he or she can truly be impartial. However, any person who is an appointed hearing officer must:

1. be independent and not be employed by the school district;
2. have no personal or professional interest that would impact negatively on his or her objectivity;
3. not have been involved in the original CSE recommendations;.
4. be certified as a hearing officer and have fulfilled all state education requirements for such a position.

The impartial hearing is an administrative procedure; it is conducted like a court proceeding with a judge (the hearing officer) and a court stenographer. The school district and the parent are represented by attorneys. The cost of legal representation is astronomical; impartial hearings can range in cost from $10,000 to $30,000, depending on the length of the hearing. Many parents who cannot pay such legal fees must seek the assistance of low-cost advocacy groups. Often these groups have long waiting lists of parents requesting their services.

The hearing procedure provides the parent and the school district with the opportunity to present arguments to determine a resolution to the dispute. The hearing process includes the calling of witnesses and cross examination by both the school district and the parent.

The hearing officer's decision will be based on the information presented during the hearing, and will include the reasons and the basis for the decision. The decision will also state that each party has the right to appeal the decision to the Commissioner of Education. Parents are always shocked to discover that they can be taken to an impartial hearing by the school district if they do not comply. A school district might request such a hearing

1. if the parent does not consent to an evaluation by the school district. The BOE can request a hearing to conduct an evaluation despite the parent's refusal.
2. if the parent requests an independent evaluation and the district refuses. The BOE may initiate an impartial hearing to resolve the dispute.
3. if the parent does not consent to the recommendation for special education. The BOE can request an impartial hearing.

Personal Insights

The due process mechanism was developed to ensure that the rights of the disabled can be protected beyond the decision making of the school district committee. Unfortunately, the structure of the due process procedure has created an adversarial system that pits school districts against families. The appeal process is not only time consuming, it is also financially exhausting. Most families cannot afford to hire an attorney for $10,000 to $20,000 for an impartial hearing.

It is truly unfortunate that parents are placed in a position where they feel that they must fight for the rights or the needs of their child. Districts have access to large expense budgets, but parents are often faced with exhausting their personal finances, giving in to the judgment of the school district, or moving out of the community. Although some cases have reached the Supreme Court and have been won by parents, the decision to enter into a long legal battle and to face an uncertain outcome is difficult.

DISABLED PRESCHOOL CHILDREN

After **PL 94-142** was passed, many researchers and educators argued that the law did not mandate services for children from birth to five years and therefore did not go far enough. Issues related to early identification and intervention focused on the dramatic needs of infants and preschoolers with disabling problems. The significance of the educational problem was highlighted by the fact that the technological advancements that enabled earlier diagnosis of many disorders did not then result in educational intervention. Services to infants and preschoolers were not mandated in educational settings and, as a result, voluntary agencies (e.g., United Cerebral Palsy, the Association for Children with Down's Syndrome, and the Association for Children with Learning Disabilities) developed and expanded to address this need. In addition, the types and levels of services varied from community to community across the United States. Some communities provided extensive services; some provided none for disabled preschool children. As an example, Nassau and Suffolk counties in New York State established a comprehensive network system of services and agencies for disabled infants and preschoolers that surpassed the systems of many other communities in the United States. Clearly, identification requires intervention but it was not until 1986 that Public Law 99-457 was passed.

PL 99-457

Essentially, **PL 99-457** addresses two groups of disabled children. It extends to the first group—disabled preschool children ages three and four—all federal requirements, rights, and protections currently applicable to school-aged disabled children (ages 5 to 21). Such requirements include individualized education plans, adherence to least restrictive environment guidelines, and due process provisions applicable to child placement decisions (Data Research, 1988).

In addition, PL 99-457 amends the Education of the Handicapped Act to develop and implement a statewide, comprehensive, coordinated, multidisciplinary, interagency program of early intervention services for disabled infants and toddlers and their families. This policy explanation is based on the substantial need

a. to enhance the development of disabled infants and toddlers and to minimize their potential for developmental delay;
b. to reduce the educational costs to our society, including our nation's schools, by minimizing the need for special education and related services after disabled infants and toddlers reach school age;
c. to minimize the likelihood of institutionalization of disabled individuals and to maximize their potential for independent living in society; and

d. to enhance the capacity of families to meet the special needs of their infants and toddlers with disabilities.

Since the passage of PL 94-142, programs have been developed to provide educational and therapeutic services to children who were either not receiving an education or were not receiving adequate services. In the reauthorization of this act the 101st Congress changed the name of the Education of the Handicapped Act to Individuals with Disabilities Education Act (IDEA). In addition, the term *handicap* was replaced with *disability*. This law was finally passed after many years of parental struggle and advocacy. Although the development of educational programs for people with disabilities addressed a critical need, it simultaneously underscored a range of related problems that also required attention and resolution. One of these issues has been and continues to be philosophical as well as pragmatic—the role of parents in education (see Chapter 2).

Preschool Procedures

In 1986, school districts became responsible for assuring the provision of special education services to eligible preschool (three- and four-year-old) children with disabling conditions. States have developed laws and regulations that apply specifically to this population and differ from those relating to disabled school-age children.

Under the requirements of the law, each local school district must establish a Committee on Preschool Special Education (CPSE). If parents of a preschool child suspect that the child has a disabling problem, they may request referral to the CPSE (see Figure 3-7). At the time of referral, the Board of Education provides the parent with a list of approved evaluation sites. The parent may choose from among these approved programs and select the site that will conduct the evaluation. This is a major change from the CSE evaluation procedure, which does not allow for parental choice. The evaluation site will then send a representative to the CPSE as a voting member to present the evaluation results. This clearly provides a mechanism for the parents' concerns and choices to be represented. Generally, the evaluator incorporates the recommendations of the parent and the family. This involves a major departure from the operation of the CSE, which does not provide any mechanism for parent representation. Although this process is an improvement over the CSE procedure, it still does not give parents a vote on the committee; it does not go far enough (see Figure 3-9). Decisions about disabled children are made by a committee; parents have not yet been recognized as partners in the educational process.

Committee on Preschool Special Education (CPSE)

With the passage of Public Law 99-457, the CPSE, like the CSE, is constituted as a multidisciplinary team that is mandated to evaluate and process children

Figure 3-7
The CPSE Process: Three to Five Years

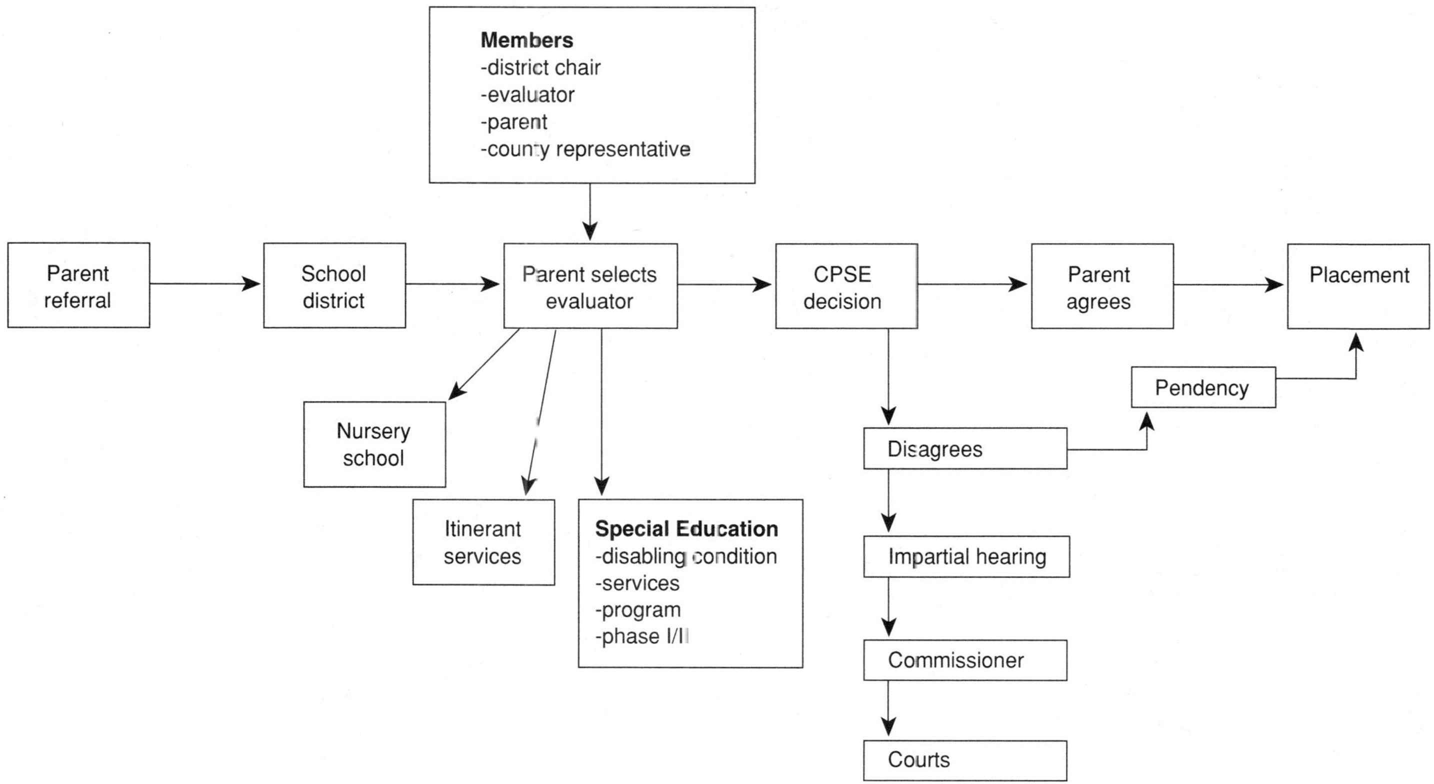

three to five years of age. If the child is eligible for special education services, the CPSE will develop a recommendation for a program and services that have been approved by the state's education department. As with school-age children, special education procedures must follow a specific time line for evaluations, meetings, and ultimate placement for the child. Preschool children with disabling conditions and their parents are entitled to all due process rights available for disabled school-age children. If the parents disagree with the decisions of the Committee on Preschool Special Education, they can request another CPSE meeting, request mediation, request an impartial hearing, and, ultimately, file legal papers for an Article 78* in court—if they have the financial resources to challenge the committee.

The Individualized Family Service Plan

The 1986 Amendment to the Education for All Handicapped Children Act, Public Law 99-457, changed the role of the family in the educational decision-making process. Within the provisions of the document is the requirement that early intervention programs providing services for infants and toddlers must develop an **Individualized Family Service Plan (IFSP)** for each child and his or her family. The **Individualized Education Program (IEP)** focuses on the needs of the *child;* the IFSP requires an analysis of *family* needs. This legislation differs from 94-142 in that services to families can be provided along with or independent of the educational needs of the disabled child. In addition, the role of the parent is quite different in the development of the IFSP. In this process the parent is a member of the multidisciplinary team that generates the educational goals and program (see Figure 3-8).

Krauss (1990) notes that the IFSP significantly alters the relationship between parent and professionals (see Figure 3-9). The newfound partnership relationship that is so explicitly described may present a problem for many professionals in early intervention programs. Although the precedent for parental participation has been established in PL 94-142, districts managing the CPSE process for three- and four-year-olds and the CSE process for children five years old and older interpret the term *participation* quite differently (Goldstein, Strickland, Turnbull, & Curry, 1980). For disabled school-age children, the Committee on Special Education (CSE) functions differently; therefore, the relationship between parent and professional is quite different. It is the mandate of the CSE to determine the child's disabling condition, to develop an Individualized Education Plan, and to place the child in the least restrictive environment. Yanok and Derubertis (1989) note that PL 94-142 has not stimulated the involvement of parents in the educational process (see Figure 3-10).

*An Article 78 is a legal proceeding by which the courts review the decisions of administrative agencies such as a state education department, causing more legal costs for parents.

Figure 3-8
Is the CPSE Process Complicated for a NEW Parent?

. . . Complication stems from the school district. If it's a "nice" district, the paperwork involved will not be so complicated. But a "not so nice" district can make the whole CPSE experience a nightmare.

. . . Yes, at first. It takes a while to become familiar with the laws, and to figure out what each party's role is in making decisions (parents, school district, preschool program).

. . . No. My experience was very easy. My son's needs were very apparent. I received all services I requested. Process did not seem complicated.

. . . Yes, it is complicated when you're dealing with it for the first time because at the same time, you're trying to understand and make decisions regarding the type of early intervention necessary and consider short- and long-term implications. You're doing this at the beginning of a learning process so you're doing it with a minimum of knowledge.

. . . I think that the answer to this question depends greatly on how cooperative your school district is. My school district was extremely helpful and I found the experience to be not too difficult.

. . . I did not find the CPSE a complicated procedure. Dialogue was basically between the school district representative and the preschool representative. Questions were directed to me. In each instance, everyone was in agreement to continue the SLCD curriculum.

. . . It can be; however, my experience with my district was that they eliminated all the confusion by communicating often and I felt that the school district wanted the best for my child.

. . . No. I feel going to parent training with Toya Davis before my actual meeting was very beneficial. Perhaps if I went to the meeting with no knowledge it could be threatening and intimidating.

. . . The CPSE process is horrible for the new parent. How is the parent supposed to know about all the rules, procedures, and regulations? How can the parent make a knowledgeable decision? Based on what? The educational system is stacked against us!

. . . Yes. The whole grading/evaluation system is very technical and clinically oriented. With much room for subjective criticism I feel the parent should be spoken to in nontechnical terms and the CPSE process as well should be clarified in the beginning so parents can plan preschool activities.

. . . Yes. Because parents who are unaware of their rights as well as unaware of their children's specific needs can get shafted during the IEP process. The chairpeople rarely explain things adequately and parents just assume that the "experts" know.

In fact, Yoshida, Fenton, Kaufman, and Maxwell (1978) indicate that school personnel noted that parents of exceptional children did not have the educational knowledge to participate in educational decision making for their children. The author suggests that parent-school partnership has not been established in many school districts due to such negative professional attitudes. With the downward extension of PL 99-457, school districts had to expand their perceptions and expectations of parent involvement. Acceptance of and respect for parental input in determining the outcome of the CPSE and ICPSE meetings are the cornerstones of a successful parent-professional relationship. This type of relationship, one based on respect and trust can only result in a win-win scenario. The family and the child win because their needs are met. The professional wins because he or she has won the respect and trust of the family.

Figure 3-9
How Would You Change the CPSE System for Families?

. . . Most families experience difficulty in the CPSE system. I think a phone hotline might help answer questions faster.

. . . School districts should have informative pre-advisory sessions with parents to explain how programming is determined. Since this is the only opportunity the parents get, both psych and speech/language pathologist should be present at CPSE to better explain to parents the testing results, not the social worker from the school that did testing.

. . . Most of the time districts have eight to ten people on CPSE. There are supposed to be four people on CPSE—the parent, the teacher or evaluator of the child, the psychologist, and the chairperson of CPSE. The parent is supposed to have a major say in what happens to the child. This should be enforced.

. . . I would like to see a family therapist available to counsel the family as a support system as well as to explain the importance of parents as advocates for their children.

. . . I feel that the on-site visit is very brief. I question the emphasis based on this information. There is no flexibility regarding the scheduled date. Two instances (the first time I was one day post-caesarean section), the school district refused to reschedule the meeting.

. . . Parents should have the option to be voting members of the CPSE.

. . . Nothing. I am very impressed with the constant communication of Rachael's teachers. I am a working, single parent with two young children in school and it's very difficult for me to be more involved in the school because of my schedule.

. . . I don't believe the school district should be involved with preschoolers. Especially those who don't believe in early intervention. The CPSE should consist of the school, parent, representative of preschool program, and appropriate physicians. Parents should be able to choose the child's educational placement.

. . . Parent training should be added in at the district level because when a child gets labeled, what does that mean. Also on the list of approved preschool providers a short blurb on the type of preschool, who it services, what kids would do best, etc.

Figure 3-10
How Would You Change the CSE Procedures?

. . . Make available a parent advocate for helping the parents though the maze of CSE. The child should be the purpose. LRE should be based on each child's needs. The state education department wants to save money and place each child in district schools rather than provide what is best for each child.

. . . Have the CSE held early to enable the parents to explore other options if they are not satisfied with the judgment (before the June date). The parents should meet with the parent advocate prior to the hearing to discuss the case.

. . . Parents should have the option to be voting members of the CSE.

. . . The procedure in place has worked for us well to date. Our school district listens to our concerns but it is clear that the district decides.

. . . I was fortunate because when I was looking for a school-age program my district gave me the list and said you visit them and decide which best meets your child's needs. When I saw SLCD I decided it was right. They said, "if that's where you want her to go that's where she'll go." I think this is how it should be. Give the parent the decision-making power; we know our children.

Parental Involvement

Federal law and regulations for the education of children with disabling conditions refer to the role of parents in the special education process in the somewhat ambiguous terms ***participation*** and ***involvement.*** It has been left to the states to interpret the federal law and to establish procedures for the participation of parents. In some states, parental involvement includes:

a. being fully informed about school programs and child rights;
b. viewing the parental role as one of partnership with the school;
c. exhibiting a willingness to become involved and interested;
d. providing support to educational programs;
e. asking questions and expressing concerns about the child's education;
f. communicating with the child about school;
g. maintaining current information on the child's educational program and progress.

The parental role does not include a voting partnership as a member of the CSE (see Figure 3-11), nor does it include decision making. It is no wonder that parents complain that their role has been trivialized by the educational process. In the last analysis, if the parents do not agree, they must initiate the next step, an impartial hearing that is adversarial and clearly aligns the parent against the school district. Aside from the tremendous financial burden, the stress and turmoil created in the family cannot even be measured. During the course of the hearing process, the child must remain in the placement indicated by the IEP (this is referred to as a pendent placement) until the dispute is resolved. Challenges to a CSE placement recommendation can be due to a variety of issues. **Pendency** can impact the placement issue either negatively or positively. For instance, if a child had been in an educational setting that was satisfactory to the parents and the CSE decides to change that placement, pendency would maintain that child in the setting until the issue was resolved. However, if a child had been in an educational setting that was not satisfactory to the parents, pendency would then maintain that unsatisfactory setting until the issue was resolved.

In most instances when impartial hearings are requested by parents, the issue is that not enough services are being provided for the child. Therefore, in most instances the child is maintained in an unsatisfactory placement. Furthermore, the school district has financial and personnel resources that parents do not. A dispute with a school district can continue for years involving time, stress, and money. Many families do not challenge the decision of the CSE because of the complications and difficulties.

Figure 3-11
Should Parents VOTE on the Committee?

. . . Yes, it's about our children.

. . . I'm not sure parents know enough about the track record and/or qualifications of the candidates on the committee to make a sound judgment.

. . . Yes, the parent should vote on the committee. The parents should involve themselves more in their children's education. All the preschools and parent organizations of school-age children should start writing state and federal representatives to serve special education. It is the time for the acorn to fall. The New Compact for Education involves doing away with all existing systems and channeling all monies into the regular education system. Good grief! Charlie Brown, take us back to the stone age! Children severely impaired will be in regular classes. They will socialize and that's all. They will have no aides—no special classes. What a great thought! Save money!! The parents must be educated to ask for their child's needs and help special education and help preschools and keep private schools open.

. . . Yes. The more active the voice, the more involved the role.

. . . Absolutely. The parent should vote on the critical issue of the child's education. As a taxpayer, I feel it is the right of the parent to choose the avenue to pursue.

. . . Maybe, depending on their education background and experience with children.

. . . Parents should have an option to vote. For a disabled child, placement, IEP, and goals affect *everyone*, including the parent and family. Therefore, a parent should have the opportunity to vote.

. . . I think this is a very gray area. Who knows what's best for the child—the parent or the system? I think you can argue both ends.

. . . Parents should have the option to be voting members of the committee. Those parents who are involved with their children's education and have acquired the knowledge necessary to cope with the disabling condition and with the committee process have given more consideration to their children's cases than the CSE/CPSE possibly could. They deserve to vote!

. . . A parent who is involved and informed with the child should be allowed to vote. I feel they have as much right to voice their opinion as anyone else at that meeting. The way it works now it makes you feel like the committee is doing you a favor. It's not. Your child is entitled to this.

. . . Yes, absolutely, unquestionably, without a doubt. As I said before, it's our children and we know them best.

Personal Insights

Originally Public Law 94-142 focused on the needs of children aged five through twenty-one. It took close to twelve years for the federal government to amend 94-142 to include infants and preschoolers. How frustrating it must have been for parents of disabled preschool children to realize after 1974 that their child was disabled but that there was no provision to educate him or her before the age of five. Many families in the United States were not in a position financially to provide educational and/or therapeutic programming for a disabled preschooler.

To realize that their children needed services that they were not able to provide motivated many parents to mobilize in the political arena. The reality of 99-457 is the reality of this frustration and anger. The amendment to 94-142 was accomplished because parents of disabled children advocated aggressively for educational support and services. Families truly represent an untapped resource in American education. Parents who are united represent a formidable coalition.

Parents need to understand the political and legislative process. They need to understand and learn how to advocate effectively for their disabled children. It is truly amazing how much most parents learn through the process of having a language disordered child. The system would work more effectively and rapidly if parents of disabled *and* nondisabled children realized their common goals and advocated together to achieve changes in education.

SUMMARY

The historical underpinnings for the passage of Public Law 94-142 involve the systematic separation of disabled individuals from all areas of American life and society. This separation had both positive and negative effects. Since 1975, special education programming has proliferated with the growing awareness of the specific needs of developmentally disabled individuals. To meet the educational needs of various populations of disabled children, a wide range of philosophical approaches, clinical procedures, therapeutic techniques, assessment tools, and programs have developed nationally. Interestingly enough, two rather striking issues have converged on the forefront of American education and present themselves as complex issues that will effect legal, procedural, and educational changes.

Mainstreaming and Inclusion

The shift away from specialized programming has been based primarily on the therapeutic argument that the integration of disabled and nondisabled children would benefit the developmentally disabled as well as the nondisabled children. The regular education class would provide disabled children with the benefit of normalized socialization experiences and interaction. Furthermore, nondisabled children would develop an acceptance and understanding of the needs of the disabled child. Proponents of mainstreaming and inclusion have argued against special, separate classes, particularly in cases where the regular education teacher could individualize the learning experience. There is also the issue that the separateness of the programming in and of itself reinforces discriminatory thinking as far as the disabled are concerned.

On the other side, researchers who support special education programming argue that mainstreaming and inclusion are not educationally appropriate for *all* disabled children. The intent of all educational legislation is not to remove the existing education options but rather to preserve them so that every disabled student is educated with appropriate services. Gottlieb (1982) states that the early research on the efficacy of special classes is no longer relevant since the population researched was mildly disabled. Whereas mainstreaming might be appropriate for the mildly disabled, moderately and severely disabled children require different alternatives than the regular classroom. Macmillan (1971) noted that the proponents of integration need to recognize that the educational profile of TMR children (trainable mentally retarded) deviates on so many academic variables that regular education is not appropriate for this group.

The idea has also been proposed that placing all disabled children in regular education classes regardless of individual needs is really a replacement of the educational system prior to the passage of Public Law 94-142—a return to an earlier time. The question becomes: Can all levels of disabled children be appropriately served in a mainstream class of thirty children? Smith and Arkans (1974) asked whether it is necessary to rediscover that a low-functioning child will become a social isolate in the regular class. Is the regular education teacher academically, educationally, and methodologically prepared to work effectively with different types of and levels of disabled children?

Many teachers and educators themselves question whether the social, personal, and emotional needs of moderately and severely retarded children can be addressed in a regular class with a teacher who is already overburdened with thirty students (Anastasiow, 1986). Warren (1979) states that the most effective type of placement for special-needs children has not yet been identified. Part of the problem is that educators and researchers are dealing with the disabled as though they represent a single, uniformed population. If education is to be successful, the concerns and needs of a group of *individuals,* not just the *group,* must be considered. The goal of special education is to prepare individuals to function in their school and their community. Quality cannot be legislated; it needs to be developed (Bishop, 1979).

Parental Choice

Parents clearly have a whole set of expectations about how the system should work, and so they are frustrated by procedural complexities and educational disillusionment as they try to negotiate through the complicated system of rules, regulations, and procedures. This is further complicated by the fact that the role of the family is clearly changing in American society. The nuclear family can no longer be defined by the working father and the mother who remains at home with two children. The multicultural demands and issues along with the increasing number of single-parent families must impact on the educational system. Parents complain that the system is procedurally complicated and confusing. They also know that at times they are being patronized by professionals in the system. It is clear that parents no longer want to settle for a secondary role in the education of their children (see Figure 3-12). The parents coming up through the family service system will not want to be relegated to a

Figure 3-12
What Should Be the Parents' Role?

. . . The most important. A parent lives with the child and knows him best.

. . . Parents have schedules (work) that must be considered for various programs. The parents should have an option for accepting the child's placement. Parents can contribute to the CPSE by sharing some personal views on their children that may not have been apparent in the rigid testing procedures.

. . . The parent does not have the right by federal law to make the decision on where the child attends, by right of fair hearing. If state education has its way of making medication mandatory, the outcome will be what State Education wants. This year we'll see. The Five Year Plan of 1988 is to bring BOCES and all children back to district. State Ed wants to do inclusion of all children into the regular classroom with an IEP in the regular classroom. They will do away with small groups and all help for children up to now.

. . . I think the parent knows the child better than anyone else and should have an active role in the decision-making process. Parents owe it to the child to find out about programs and services available in their districts.

. . . The parents are a vital part of the process. They initially recognize the need for intervention. What they lack in formal education and vernacular is compensated for by valuable information known only to the parents regarding their child.

. . . I think that the evaluation plays an important part; however, the bottom line is that parents know their children better than any evaluator. Further, I believe that test results don't reveal the true level of the child; other factors such as their ability to function in a group setting, separation handling, etc., all need to be discussed.

Some parents know enough to contribute to a CPSE or a CSE discussion while many others don't. The parents' own knowledge is what will guarantee inclusion in the CSE process. Parents should have done their homework before coming to a committee meeting, know where they are heading, and be prepared to justify their conclusions. It is the most knowledgeable parents who wield the greatest influence in the child's placement.

. . . Parents know their children better than anyone. A placement decision should be made mutually.

. . . After preschool, the parent doesn't have much decision in the child's education, only if the district disagrees with the parent does the parent have the power to make things more "complicated." A well-informed parent should and wants to contribute in the discussion. They might be able to contribute valuable information to help in the decision process. Who's to say who knows what's best for the child?

. . . I have always felt that a parent should play a major part in their child's placement. A parent coming from your training session surely knows enough to contribute valuable insights into their child's educational needs. However, from serving as the parent representative on my school district CSE/CPSE I am appalled at the limited knowledge parents have. There are some who blindly put their faith into the school district educators, and there are MANY parents who don't even show up for their child's annual CSE review and placement.

. . . While the parent is not qualified to make a technical evaluation of the child's progress and needs, he/she does see the short- and long-term results of each program, and knows whether the child is comfortable and happy or not. Therefore, the parents can make *some* contribution to the meetings.

. . . The parents' role is minimal. Once your child is identified as a potential problem you are able to select the site where he/she is evaluated. Very often you don't find out the results of the evaluation until the CPSE meeting. But if a parent wants to become involved in education and feels they are capable of deciding, then by all means they should decide.

nonvoting role on a CSE (Committee on Special Education). In the next chapter, the changing role of the family will be discussed and this issue will be further highlighted, but it is clear that mainstreaming and parental involvement will create procedural changes in education during the upcoming decade. The form that special education will take in the future clearly is evolving and changing. If we consider the history of minority groups and their struggle to gain equal rights, we recognize that it is a process. Although African Americans were given the right to vote in 1870, it wasn't until the civil rights legislation of the 1960s that they were given access to equal education, housing, and employment. Women were assured the right to vote in 1920; however, today they are still advocating for an equal rights amendment to ensure equal educational and employment opportunities (Stuckless & Castle, 1979). The history of our country and its legislation of equal rights demonstrates that it is a process and that the process involves challenge, litigation, and strong advocacy. It is only through this process that the intent of PL 94-142 and PL 99-457 will be achieved.

A Few Words from Toya Davis

My name is Toya Davis and I am a parent of a special-needs child, Jonathan. It has been a long and difficult process for me and my family with Jonathan but we have all learned a great deal about the educational experience. I feel that it is important for professionals to understand the road that parents travel as they come to terms with a difficult realization. My child is different and has special learning needs. I have come to see in my own experience with other parents that the ability to accept the child allows the family to move forward. It is my purpose here to provide some insights into my personal experience so that teachers and therapists can better understand the internal process for many parents of disabled children. Finally, perhaps the greatest realization for me has involved the connection between Jonathan's growth and my own. I have gained a great deal from learning about Jonathan. The reality is that my son taught me many things about myself and life in general.

After having read all of the evaluations completed on Jonathan (i.e., language and communication evaluation, psychological evaluation, movement evaluation, and occupational therapy evaluation) it was decision making time. When I decided to enroll Jonathan in a local preschool program, I had absolutely no idea about the procedural process. In 1984, preschool special education was not mandated by federal law. In New York State, for example, disabled children from birth to age five could receive services by petitioning Family Court in their local communities. Since Jonathan was three years old at the time of evaluation, I had the extraordinary opportunity to choose not only the evaluation site but also the program. As a parent of a disabled child, I visited many different preschool programs, observed classrooms, and asked questions. I learned a great deal about various therapeutic populations, services, clinical techniques, educational procedures, and, most important, philosophical perspectives. I felt that as Jonathan's parent I had the right and the role to decide about his education. I took my responsibility quite seriously. I literally developed a programmatic analysis that assisted in my decision making. Given the severity of Jonathan's language disorder, I chose the School for Language and Communication Development. I therefore initiated the process by signing the Family Court petition, which was forwarded to the Nassau County Department of Mental Health for educational and procedural review. DMH then sent the petition to Family Court for jurisdictional approval. The school and my family were then notified that the program and its services were appropriate to meet Jonathan's needs; a start date was arranged along with busing and Jonathan began his educational career as a preschooler.

For the next two years Jonathan and I went to school. The educational facility generated an IEP that delineated his annual goals for each of his therapeutic services (occupational therapy, dance-movement therapy, music therapy, auditory training, and language therapy) and the classroom. It was a safe, nurturing, and supportive experience for Jonathan and for me. The both of us were learning and I knew that I would take these skills with me for the rest of my life. When Jonathan turned five, I and hundreds of other parents faced a very different kind of procedural experience. In fact, as I watched many other parents proceed through the CSE process, I realized how unfair the system was for parents of disabled children. In my own case, I was lucky. I resided in a local school district whose CSE chairperson included me in the process of educational decision making and placement. My shock and horror grew as I listened to the agonies of parents I had known for the past two years. Parents in different school districts were not given the same respect and support that I had received. I learned sadly the realities of PL 94-142. The disabled child's educational future is voted on and decided by a committee that does not include me, the parent. In essence, this committee could technically make a decision—placement and services—without me. Even if I felt that the decision concerning my child was wrong, I could only challenge the committee if I could afford—emotionally and financially—a long-term legal battle: another CSE meeting, mediation, impartial hearing, appeal to the Commissioner, State Supreme Court, U.S. Supreme Court. During this arduous battle, my Jonathan would remain in the district's placement. What an agony it would be to watch my child go through all of this, and I could only "do what I could afford to do."

The school age rules and procedures were the exact opposite of the preschool ones that I had experienced. I was no longer the decision maker; my participation was reduced to trivial lip service. In 1986, my thought was "thank God I had the preschool experience." PL 99-457 was passed to ensure disabled preschool children a free and appropriate education, but, to my dismay, the school age rules were rolled down.

In 1989, I, with many other parents, fought in New York State to protect the rights of parents of disabled preschool children. Although Jonathan was now enrolled in a school-age program in my district, I felt a strong sense of commitment to parents of disabled preschool children who were now themselves beginning the process. I therefore worked to mobilize other parents not only to fight for their rights but also to ensure that New York State established a preschool system that would incorporate the rights that I had had the privilege of experiencing with Jonathan. There were several issues that I felt were important to me as a parent of disabled children.

First, the right to *choose* my child's program had to be protected. I did not feel that any parent should be alienated and disenfranchised by a committee's decision. My relationship with my child involves my ability as a parent to be a decision maker. Since these rules for disabled preschool children were part of a federal entitlement, the parent's perception of the process became very important. If parents were frightened by the system they would not put their three- or four-year-old in school. Clearly the system had to work very differently; families had to be nurtured and supported. The parent had to play a significant role in decision making and, clearly, that could not just be lip service. The second issue was that a number of voluntary programs had existed for many, many years providing services for disabled preschool children. New York State, particularly the State Education Department, did not have a right to dismantle an effective network system to force families into local school districts. I had learned early on that this network system included highly specialized programs that met the needs of specific disabled populations. The local school district could not possibly provide the services that United Cerebral Palsy could provide. The local school district did not have the background, the experience, or the commitment to a cerebral palsied child that UCP had. New York State, unlike most states, already had a system in place; this system of preschool programs should be recognized and incorporated into any system created by the state. If children, their rights, and their education were the first priority here, the programs that had served those children in the past were the best programs to continue meeting their needs.

As a parent of a disabled child, I was learning not only about Jonathan but about the political process that established procedures for educational development. Networking with other parents in 1989, I truly learned about empowerment. I met legislators, educators, and other parents. The system could only work and can only work with empowered parents. No one could do for Jonathan what I did, and only a system that included me in the process could have me as a contributor. I had come a long way since Jonathan was three years old. I had walked a very difficult road and now I saw my path as one that helped other parents through the process.

REFERENCES

Anastasiow, N. (1986). The research base for early intervention. *Journal of the Division for Early Childhood, 10,* 99–105.

Balla, D. (1976). Relationship of institution size to quality of care: A review of the literature. *American Journal of Mental Deficiency, 81,* 117–124.

Bishop, M. (1979). Mainstreaming: A goal or a process? In M. Bishop (Ed.), *Mainstreaming: Practical ideas for educating hearing-impaired students.* Washington, DC: The Alexander Graham Bell Association for the Deaf.

Bloom, B. (1964). *Stability and change in human characteristics.* New York: John Wiley.

Butterfield, E. C. (1967). The role of environmental factors in the treatment of institutionalized mental retardates. In A. A. Baumerster (Ed.), *Mental retardation: Appraisal, education and rehabilitation.* Chicago: Aldine.

Data Research, Inc. (1988). *Handicapped students and special education,* 5th ed. Rosemount, MN: Data Research, Inc.

Dublinske, S. (1989). Children with communication disorders: Public policy issues. *Journal of Childhood Communication Disorders, 12,* 119–126.

Hageny, W. (1986). School law—1986: A handbook for school board members. New York State School Boards Association, Inc., Washington Avenue, Albany, NY.

Healy, A., Keesee, P., & Smith, B. (1989). Early services for children with special needs: Transactions for family support. Iowa City: University Hospital School.

Hunt, J. (1961). *Intelligence and experience.* New York: Ronald.

Kirk, S. (1958). *Early education of the mentally retarded.* Urbana, IL: University of Illinois Press.

Krauss, M. W. (1990). New precedent in family policy: Individualized family service plan. *Exceptional Children, 56,* 388–395.

Marozas, D. S., & May, D. C. (1988). *Efficacy issues and practices in special education.* White Plains, NY: Longman.

Mayer, C. L. (1982). *Educational administration and special education: A handbook for school administrators.* Boston: Allyn and Bacon.

Meisels, S. (1985). The efficacy of early intervention: Why are we still asking this question? *Topics in Early Childhood Special Education, 5,* 1–11.

Palmer, F. (1977). The effects of early childhood intervention. Paper presented at the Annual Meeting of the American Association for the Advancement of Science, Denver, CO.

A parent's guide to special education. (March 1990). Albany, NY: University of the State of New York, State Education Department.

Rosetti, L. (1986). High-risk infants: Identification, assessment, and intervention. Boston: A College Hill Publication.

Sarason, S. (1982). *The culture of the school and the problem of change.* Boston: Allyn and Bacon.

Skeels, H. (1966). Adult status of children with contrasting early life experiences. Monograph of the Society for Research in Child Development, 31.

Stuckless, R., & Castle, W. (1979). The law and its implications for mainstreaming. In M. Bishop (Ed.), *Mainstreaming: Practical ideas for educating hearing-impaired students.* Washington, DC: The Alexander Graham Bell Association for the Deaf.

Warren, S. (1979). What is wrong with mainstreaming? A comment on drastic change. *Mental Retardation, 17,* 301–303.

Yanok, J. (1986). Free appropriate public education for handicapped children: Congressional intent and judicial interpretation. *Remedial and Special Education, 7,* 49–53.

Yanok, J., & Derubertis, D. (1989). Comparative study of parental participation in regular and special education programs. *Exceptional Children,* 195–199.

Yoshida, R. K., Fenton, K. S., Kaufman, M. J., & Maxwell, J. P. (1978). Parental involvement in special education pupil planning process: The school's perspective. *Exceptional Children, 44,* 531–534.

Zigler, E. (1973). The retarded child as a whole person. In D. K. Routh (Ed.), *The experimental psychology of mental retardation.* Chicago: Aldine.

CHAPTER

4

EARLY IDENTIFICATION AND ASSESSMENT

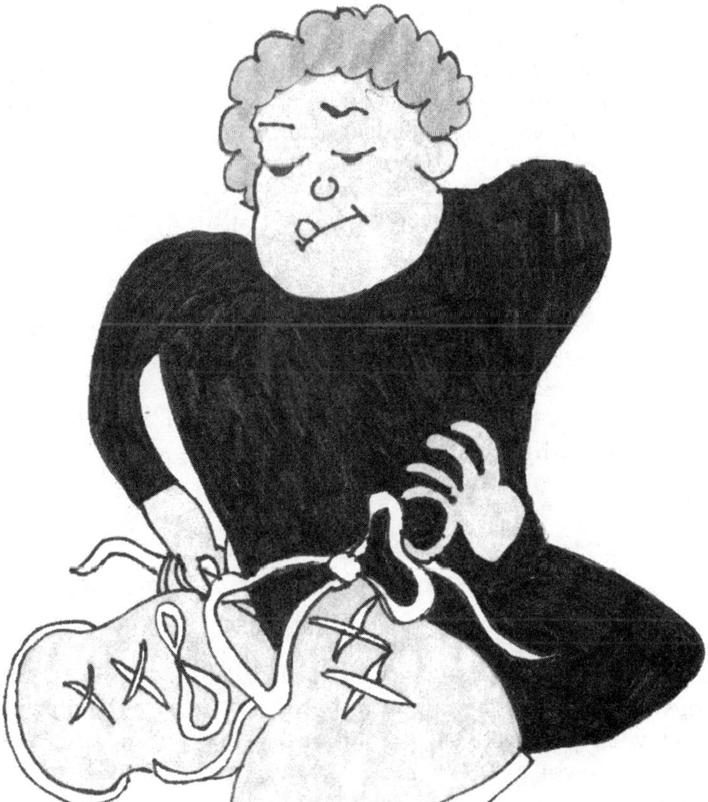

Public Law 99-457 extended the federal requirements, rights, and protections previously available only to school-aged disabled children downward to include preschool children and infants birth to age five. The impact of this legislation is monumental. Previously, diagnostic teams focused on the child. With this extension, a more encompassing ecological perspective became necessary in order to serve the child under the age of five. Within the framework of this law the professional skills of the speech/language pathologist are invaluable for speech-delayed youngsters and their families. The pathologist is skilled in assessing the communicative speech language behaviors of the child and the communicative interactions of the parents/caregivers, and can provide insights into enhancing and developing communication skills. For the young child most early learning is mediated through language; therefore, it is vital that speech-impaired children and their families participate in an intervention program with the speech/language pathologist (SLP).

Public Law 99-457 required an Individual Education Plan (IEP) for children three to five years of age. Generally, this plan centered on the needs of the child. Parental input was considered and the Committee for Preschool Special Education generated an IEP that was acceptable to the family. Part H of PL 99-457 calls for an Individualized Family Service Plan (IFSP) for children from birth through two years. This IFSP focuses on the needs of the family as well as the needs of the child. For instance, if a parent needs counseling in order to function more appropriately with the disabled infant/toddler, the IFSP will include such counseling. If a parent has economic hardship and has no means of getting to the counseling services, the IFSP will provide for transportation. The philosophy that generated PL 99-457 and supports this approach to serving disabled children is that the needs of the child and the needs of the family are intertwined and interdependent. Meeting family needs is necessary in order to meet the needs of the child.

This chapter will focus on questions such as: What constitutes early identification and assessment for the young preschool child and infant? What assessment techniques, strategies, and instruments are suitable for this assessment process? Who is being evaluated and assessed? What is being evaluated and assessed? In addition, other issues will be considered, such as culturally different populations and at-risk issues.

The Journey Begins

The official journey to assessing and identifying the communicatively disabled youngster begins with a phone call. But even before the parent makes that initial contact with the professional, he or she has already considered carefully the functioning level of the child. Generally, parents state that they have felt for

This chapter was authored by Dr. Christine Radziewicz.

months that the child has not acquired age-appropriate communication skills. However, their initial questionings have usually been quieted by statements from friends, spouses, parents, and, occasionally, even professionals that the child will outgrow these delays, that time will take care of it. In fact, once a child has been identified as communicatively disabled, parents often ask how long it will take the child to catch up or to outgrow the delay. Parents are eager for answers immediately because they have been filled with doubts for some time.

The initial parent-professional contact should be informative, clear, and unhurried. The parents need to know the steps involved in assessing the preschool child. They need to know the types of evaluations performed, the time framework, and the possible outcomes before any initial appointments at the evaluation center are even scheduled. The evaluation process is a somewhat lengthy and difficult one for the family and the child. Consider the following as a possible procedure to follow once the assessment journey begins.

The mother calls the diagnostic center and indicates that her child is not communicating or speaking as well as other children. She is connected to a professional who will listen and reinforce the appropriateness of the parent's call and the probable need for assessing the child. The professional to whom the mother first speaks is often the speech/language pathologist, who is certainly qualified to answer questions regarding the child's communication behaviors and will be one of the members of the transdisciplinary team that interviews the parents and evaluates the child.

There has been an explosion of information regarding the communication behaviors of children from birth through five since the passage of PL 99-457 in 1986. In 1990, the American Speech Language Association published a position statement on the role of speech/language pathologists in service delivery to infants, toddlers, and their families. This position statement clarifies the roles and responsibilities of the SLP as including:

a. screening and identification;
b. assessment and evaluation;
c. the design, planning, direct delivery, and monitoring of treatment programs;
d. case management;
e. consultation with and referral to agencies and other professionals providing services to this young population and their families.

> These roles should be assumed in a comprehensive community-based program that is family-centered and is also coordinated with other services that the families and their children may need or receive. The speech/language pathologist should be an integral member of any multidisciplinary team serving families and their infants or toddlers (ASHA, 1990).

It becomes clear from this position statement that the speech/language pathologist is integral to the identification and remediation of the speech-impaired infant and preschooler.

At the time of the initial contact with the family, the parent should be assured that he or she acted in a responsible manner and is an important component in determining the needs of the child. Further information can then be provided, including an overview of the kind and number of appointments to be scheduled and the time framework in which these appointments will take place. After all questions have been carefully answered, the parent is given the option to schedule an initial appointment or to wait and consider all of the information presented and call later—either to ask more questions or to schedule an appointment. Generally, parents feel comfortable enough to schedule the first appointment at that time because some of their fears and doubts have been answered.

The Process of Family-Focused Assessment

In order to understand the process of child assessment it is necessary to consider the process and how it has evolved over time. Before the passage of Public Law 94-142, parents played only a minor role in planning the educational programming for their disabled children. However, PL 94-142 mandated parental participation in the planning of the individualized education plan of a child of five years or older, and set mechanisms in place to resolve disagreements between parents and educational institutions (due process rights). Passage of PL 94-142 was the beginning of parent involvement; over time this component took on different features. When Public Law 99-457 made assessment and appropriate education an entitlement for preschool children from birth to five years, it became evident that with the preschool population involved, parents must be integral constituents of the educational process.

Figure 4-1
Ecological Perspective

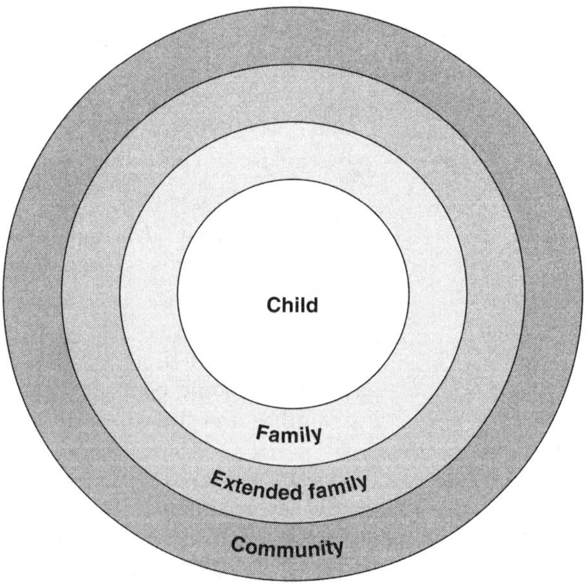

Because the parent is the front-line service provider and edu preschool child, what has evolved is a change in focus from assessing and strengths of the disabled child to assessing the needs and strengths of the child *and the family.* This enlarged view of the child as part of a family system (Bell, 1968) encouraged the genesis of an ecological view of development. Bronfenbrenner (1977) expanded and conceptualized this ecological view to consider the child as a member of a family unit, which in turn is a member of a larger community. The concentric circles in Figure 4-1 attempt to show this ecological perspective. This view challenges the traditional approach of the child-focused assessment process, which was authoritarian and therapy intensive and focused on deficit functioning.

A complete assessment of a young child requires a team of professionals to determine whether or not the child demonstrates age-appropriate development in the areas of cognition, communication, motor skill development, physical development, and social emotional development.

TEAM MODELS AND OUTCOMES

There are three types of team assessment models. In the **multidisciplinary team model,** which is frequently utilized in medical settings, several different professionals assess. Each works independently, but important information is shared. Treatment goals are planned in isolation of the other disciplines. In the **interdisciplinary team model,** different professionals assess, then exchange information. Although treatment goals may be jointly planned, delivery of services is often isolated. In the **transdisciplinary team model,** different professionals work together across discipline boundaries, with the purpose of integrating their findings into a transdisciplinary treatment plan. This model of assessment and intervention is considered most appropriate for families and children. PL 99-457 identified professionals from ten disciplines as possible members of the team—an audiologist, a speech/language pathologist, an early childhood special educator, an occupational therapist, a physical therapist, a physician, a social worker, a nurse, a nutritionist, and a psychologist. Not all ten professionals need participate in the multidisciplinary team; the needs of the family and the child determine the necessary members of the team. Cooperation among all team members is of paramount importance. Inherent in this model is interdependence among team members; each member can attain his or her goals only if the other team members achieve theirs. In addition, all team members must have thorough knowledge of infant development, assessment procedures, and intervention techniques (McCollum & Hughes, 1988). For example, consider the disabled child who is cared for by a grandparent. The social worker has ascertained from interview and needs assessment that the mother of the child is anxious because the child does not relate to her as well as to the grandmother. One goal that the social worker prioritizes is decreasing the mother's anxiety. The SLP has ascertained through her assessment that this child does not have imitation skills and that the parent-infant interaction between mother and child is somewhat mismatched; that is, the mother does not utilize physical proximity or eye gaze to keep the child interactive and interested. Utilizing a transdisciplinary approach, the SLP and the social worker must integrate their findings and develop a common strategy of intervention that meets the needs of the mother and the needs of the child. Rather than initially focus on the communicative behaviors/interactions between the grandmother and the mother, the SLP will focus on the interactions between the mother and the child. Mother could be shown how to increase the length, number, and diversity of social interactions. Playing games such as "this little piggy" or "peek-a-boo" would develop more appropriate eye gaze patterns between the mother and the child, encourage imitation in the child, and enhance the overall pleasure of mother-child interactions.

Team management—the way a team performs its duties—is of central importance to a transdisciplinary team. The team that works well together makes a variety of decisions and shares the responsibility of those decisions. One member is chosen to be the coordinator or manager; he or she is generally someone with whom the parents have a comfortable and trusting relationship and whose expertise relates to the child's area of disability. The most likely team manager in the case of the child with a suspected speech language delay, for example, would be the SLP, who was probably the first professional with whom the parent spoke and was probably the first to meet the family and the child. The information gained from the family would be utilized by the SLP to decide which other members of the team should assess the child, such as the psychologist, the early childhood special educator, or the occupational therapist. The team would then pool all the information that was gained through observation, interview, and test data, and reach a decision for additional assessments, intervention, or reevaluation. This information and recommendation would be shared and discussed with the family.

Individualized Family Service Plan

The outcome of a transdisciplinary assessment of a child under the age of three is the Individualized Family Service Plan (IFSP); for a child three to five years old, it is an Individualized Education Plan (IEP). The IFSP is similar to the IEP; however, the focus of the IEP is the child, while the focus of the IFSP is the child and the family. Specifically, the IFSP provides information regarding the child's current level of functioning, family strengths, family needs, specific program services (such as frequency and intensity), date of initiation, and anticipated duration. It is important that the IFSP include the changes the family wants for their child and/or themselves. The IFSP should not be full of professional jargon. It should be clear and its goals should be understood not only by the professionals who participated in the assessment but by the parents as well. Chapter 3 provides more detailed information regarding the IEP and the CPSE.

FAMILY ASSESSMENT

In order for an assessment to be complete, the team must acknowledge the importance of the family and conduct a family-focused assessment, in which both family and professionals consider the child in the family. Traditionally only the needs and strengths of the child were considered; now the needs and strengths of the family must be brought to the forefront. When family strengths are considered, parents feel competent; when family needs are met, they feel empowered.

The family assessment is inclusive of the child's strengths and needs. It interfaces community institutions with parents in order to enhance a family's ability to function well and to facilitate development of the disabled child (Weiss, 1988). The family assessment model meets the challenge of implementation of Part H of PL 99-457, which directs agencies to support and enable parents to be aware of and choose from a wide range of creative intervention options for themselves and their children (Soper, 1991). PL 99-457 was designed to determine the resources, priorities, and concerns of the family related to enhancing the development of the child.

Factors to Consider

Several factors must be considered when shifting the focus from child-centered assessment to family assessment. One must remember that although assessment of the disabled infant is assured through law, it is up to the family to decide if they want an assessment to be performed. If the family understands that they are respected by the professional team and that their needs as well as their child's needs are considered important, they are more likely to be committed to the assessment process. The assessment must be conducted by personnel trained to utilize appropriate methods and procedures and is based on information provided by the family through a personal interview. The assessment must incorporate the family's description of its resources, priorities, and concerns.

Several important questions need to be considered before the assessment process begins: What strategies should be used in this assessment process? When is the best time for a family assessment to be done? How can the team prevent the family from viewing the assessment process as intrusive? Who should perform the family assessment? What if the team identifies a family need that the family does not recognize? Why is an assessment of family strengths important?

With these questions in mind, it becomes clear that the following are characteristics of an effective family assessment.

- It is conducted in a manner that is positive for families.
- It recognizes that family values and traditions are important.
- It includes key family members.
- It is nonintrusive.
- It targets the needs and resources of the family.

Dunst and Trivette (1988) suggest a model for a family systems assessment. Their model focuses on the family and they compare the family systems approach to the operation of a touring bike. The touring bike utilizes many gears, and even though one gear may play the most important role at a specific moment, it is the smooth alignment among all gears that generates momentum. They liken the gears to the needs, aspirations, strengths, support, and resources of the family. The momentum of the touring bike is influenced by terrain, just as the momentum of the family is affected by the developmental course of the family. If the family's needs, aspirations, strengths, resources, and support all come into play in a timely manner, the family can overcome a difficult course and gain momentum and energy—just as the touring bike can overcome a difficult terrain when the gears are aligned and operating optimally. Keep in mind that the goal of a family systems assessment is the identification of the "gears" that will propel the family and generate the energy it needs to function optimally. The assessment team's goal is *not* to define the family and take control; rather it is to help the family members define themselves and take control of the family's developmental course. How can the assessment team facilitate this empowerment of the family, and how does this empowerment benefit the disabled child? Dunst and Trivette (1988) propose four assessment goals and highlight the relationship of these goals to outcome. Consideration of their goals and outcomes will answer these two important questions. The outcome of identifying family aspirations through utilization of needs-based assessment procedures is positive child-, parent-, and family-functioning through intervention efforts that focus on these family identified needs. The outcome of identifying family strengths and capabilities is an enhancement of successful efforts in meeting family needs. The outcome of mapping the family's personal social network is an assurance of the availability and adequacy of resources based on the family's strong personal social network. The outcome of enabling the family to become more competent in mobilizing resources is an increased ability of the family to be more self-sustaining as regards its needs.

There are multiple dimensions to be considered in a family assessment. These include parent-child interactions; the parents' sense of competence, feelings of stress, and acceptance of the disabled child; sibling relationships; needs of the family; the family's support network; and the family's coping style. The assessment team can utilize tests, survey instruments, rating scales, observations, and interviews to determine family dimensions. The team must recognize that each family is unique, that family needs change over time, and that the family is embedded insociety.

Assessment Instruments

There are available a variety of formal family assessment instruments; see Table 4-1 for a sampling.

The purpose of these instruments is to measure areas such as stress, support, and parent interaction in families; they are usually administered by a professional such as a social worker or a psychologist. In addition to administering these scales/questionnaires, this professional must also have other basic skills. Bailey (1987) recommends that the personnel possess an understanding of family from a systems perspective, use effective listening and interviewing techniques, negotiate values and priorities to provide quality services to children, and be able to function as case managers in order to match family needs with community resources.

Another area of assessment that is of paramount importance to the speech/language pathologist is parent-child interaction. Previous research (Bell & Harper, 1977; Brazelton, 1982; Lewis & Rosenblum, 1974; Tronick & Ganino, 1986) has identified parent-child social interactions as bidirectional and homeostatic. That is, during a communicative interaction between parent and child, each is an active member of the interaction, and each makes adaptations to the other's behavior. When the infant is very young the parent facilitates organization of the child's behavior and bears most of the responsibility for the interaction. As the child becomes older, he or she shares more responsibility for the interaction and learns to interact in a communicative style that matches the style of the parent. In optimal circumstances, there is a good fit or matching

Table 4-1
Family Assessment Instruments

Assessment Instrument	Publicher/Source
Critical Events Checklist (Bailey, et al., 1986)	*Journal of Early Childhood, 10*(2), 156–171.
Family Support Scale (Dunst & Jenkins, 1983)	Western Carolina Center Morganton, NC 28655
Parenting Stress Index (PSI) (Abidin, 1983)	Pediatric Psychology Press 2915 Idlewood Drive Charlottesville, VA 22901
Survey of Family Needs (Bailey & Simeonsson, 1985)	Families Project Frank Porter Graham Child Development Center University of North Carolina Chapel Hill, NC 27514

and parent-child interchanges are pleasant and sustaining (Thomas & Chess, 1977). Since these early parent-child interactions lay the foundation for further speech language learning, it is imperative that the SLP be skilled in assessing them. Assessment can be through observation and use of a parent-child interaction scale. There are several assessment instruments available. See Table 4-2 for a list of several that would be useful to the SLP.

It should be noted that proper use of these scales requires a videotape recorder, a camera, and a playback monitor. These scales are effective in identifying strengths and weaknesses in the parent-child interactive dyad. This information enables the speech/language pathologist to work with the family in understanding their own interactive style as well as that of their child. Highlighting the behaviors that enhance communication empowers parents to become more effective teachers, models, and communication partners. The speech/language pathologist is particularly equipped to work with parents to enhance communicative styles and strategies. The SLP's educational training background includes familiarity with areas such as prespeech, language, play, social routines, gestures, intentions, and parent-child interactions.

All of the information gained from observations, interviews, and parent-infant assessment scales can readily be translated into intervention goals by the SLP. Recently, Crais and Roberts (1991) developed a decision-making framework for early intervention that they refer to as decision trees. This framework is appropriate for children three months to five years and is an alter-

Table 4-2
Parent-Child Interaction Assessments

Assessment Instrument	Publisher/Source
Social Interaction Assessment/Intervention	
Assesses communicative social interaction between the parent and the disabled child (useful for children 2–34 months).	McCollum (1984). *Child: Care, Health and Development, 10,* 301–315. McCollum & Stayton (1985). *Journal of the Division for Early Childhood, 9 (2),* 125–135.
Interaction Rating Scales	
Assesses the parent's imitating, affect, gaze pattern, dyadic reciprocity, and interaction style.	Clark & Siefer (1985). *Infant Mental Health Journal, 6,* 214–225.
Teaching Skills Inventory	
Assesses the parents' verbal instructions and the child's interest level during interactions (useful for children 2–36 months)	Rosenberg, Robinson, & Beckman (1984). *Journal of the Division for Early Childhood, 8,* 107–113.
Parent/Caregiver Involvement Scale	
Assesses 11 adult behaviors during play interactions with the child (useful for children 2–57 months)	Farran, Kasari, Yoder, Harber, Huntington, & Comfort-Smith (1987). In T. Tamer (Ed.), *Stimulation and intervention in infant development.* London: Freund Publishing.

native to standardized testing. The decision trees include a sequenced set of questions followed by available response choices; they assess social interaction, comprehension, and production, and have been recommended as guidelines for assessment and management by Yoder and Kent (1988). This highly organized framework is very convenient and suitable for the SLP who is assessing and working with young children who are speech-disabled. It is designed for disabled and at-risk children with the understanding that many children receiving early intervention services may be chronologically older than three years, but developmentally in the three-month to three-year age range.

Figure 4-2 represents a social interaction tree and a comprehension tree for a child at the one-word utterance stage.

The Association for the Care of Children's Health (1988) defined a family-centered service delivery model as one in which the family is recognized as the constant in the child's life with service systems recognized as temporary and fluctuating. Parents and professionals who collaborate and participate in a partnership respect each other and are committed to each other. Professionals must share complete information with parents about their child; must implement policies and programs that provide emotional and financial support to meet the needs of the family; and must recognize family strengths and respect the family's coping mechanism. The needs of the disabled child as well as the needs of the whole family must be considered when developing intervention plans. Parents have valuable information to share with other parents and are a source of strength to each other. Clearly this model incorporates interrelatedness between families and professionals. At the policy level and at the service level the family is the focal point.

The speech/language pathologist must be familiar with family assessment instruments and must be ready to function in a collaborative fashion with the family. One of the tenets of PL 99-457 Part H is that a service coordinator be in place to work with the family, help coordinate all services, and participate in the development of the Individualized Family Service Plan (IFSP). The service coordinator is chosen by the family and, in the case of the speech-impaired child, may very well be the speech/language pathologist.

CHILD ASSESSMENT

Child assessment is best achieved through both formal and informal assessment techniques. Formal assessment instruments are either standardized norm-referenced instruments or standardized criterion-referenced instruments. Norm-referenced tests compare a single child's performance to a representative sample of the performance of other children of the same age. Norm-referenced tests must be valid and reliable and can render scores in the form of developmental age scores, developmental quotients, standard scores, and percentile ranks. Criterion-referenced tests measure a child's performance

Figure 4-2

Decision Tree for a Child at the One-Word Utterance Stage

SOCIAL INTERACTION*

	Assessment Questions	If YES	If NO	*Intervention Activities*
1	Does child verbally exhibit any earlier developing intentions (i.e., attention-seeking, requests, protests) with familiar people?	YES	NO	Go to Decision Tree for child at the prelinguistic stage.
2	Does child nonverbally exhibit any intentions with unfamiliar people?	YES	NO	Attempt to elicit attention by bringing out novel or action toys (e.g., windup toy). After demonstrating toy, allow it to stop, and reinforce any signal from child indicating interest.
3	Does child verbally exhibit any intentions with unfamiliar person?	YES	NO	Use "reported" verbally expressed intentions (e.g., "no") and play a game where at each turn child can respond "no" (e.g., offer wrong puzzle pieces). Begin by modeling and then wait for child's response.
4	Does child verbally express a variety of communicative intentions?	YES	NO	During daily activities or play routines create a need for communication and model utterances to express a child's intentions, (e.g., build a block tower and say "more block" when need another and "block fall" when tower falls).
5	Does child initiate a familiar play routine related to the context and then take one turn in the interaction?	YES	NO	Set up environment to encourage a familiar routine (e.g., position yourself for a tickle routine) and pause for child's turn. If no response, model approximate initiation (e.g., "tickle").
6	Does child maintain attention to a play activity or interaction for a continuous minute, when playing with a "focused" adult?	YES	NO	Select activity or game (e.g., pat-a-cake, horsie) the child enjoys and plays for an increasingly longer period of time, maintaining child's attention.
7	Does child take turns in an interaction by exchanging social roles during game (e.g., adult tickles child, then child becomes the "tickler")?	YES	NO	Play familiar game and model the initiator's role for the child (e.g., take child's hands and tickle yourself).
8	Does child participate in play routines associated with daily activities (e.g., rubber duck jumps into bath and quacks at start of each bath time)?	YES	NO	Begin repeating the same action or action/sound sequence at the same time during a daily activity.
9	Does child take three turns in an interaction or in a play activity initiated by an adult?	YES	NO	Initiate a play activity or interaction (e.g., pat-a-cake, peek-a-boo), pause for child's response (e.g., with hands ready to clap), take another turn quickly (e.g., clap) and pause again.

*As the child's communicative skills improve, these turn-taking behaviors should first be seen vocally and later verbally.

Figure 4-2
Continued

COMPREHENSION

	Assessment Questions		*Intervention Activities*
1	Does child respond to common routines when contextual clues are not present (e.g., "Let's go bye-bye")?	NO	Go to Decision Tree for child at the prelinguistic stage.
	YES		
2	Does child respond to any two-word sequences (e.g., kiss baby, eat cookie)?	NO	Choose object familiar to child and select one common action (e.g., eat, drink). Play games acting on and labeling the object and action.
	YES		
3	Does child respond to a variety of semantic relations in two-word utterances using familiar words (e.g., agent + action, possessor + object, or action + object: e.g., "horse eat," "dog bite")?	NO	Select words in child's one-word comprehension vocabulary. Label, and act out different combinations (e.g., "boy eat," "baby's shoe," "throw toy").
	YES		
4	Can child respond to a variety of semantic relations in two-word utterances with less familiar combinations (e.g.,"horse sit," "dog kiss")?	NO	Play games using and labeling different objects with same action, and different actions with same object.
	YES		
5	Does child respond to one action + one object requests (e.g.,"kiss baby")?	NO	Start with familiar actions on objects (e.g., eat cookie, throw ball) then move to less familiar actions (e.g., pat ball).
	YES		
6	Does child respond to 2 two-part sequences, for example, 1 action + 2 objects (e.g., "push the ball and block"), or 2 actions + 1 object (e.g., "kiss the dolly and hug dolly")?	NO	Select agent and action words in child's comprehension vocabulary. Target initially agent + action "baby eat" and action + object "eat cookie" sequences. Act out and label (e.g., "kiss baby" and then "hug baby" while playing with doll).
	YES		
7	Does child respond approximately to simple *wh* questions (e.g., what, where, who)?	NO	Ask *wh* questions in social games (e.g., "where is your nose, ears?" and model response, "Here's my nose.") Repeat question and response. Start with "what," then "who," and "where."
	YES		

Source: Crais, E., and Leonard, R. (1991). Decision making in assessment and early intervention planning. *Language, Speech, and Hearing Services in Schools, 22,* 19–30.

on a predetermined set of skills that relate either to academic performance or to daily living (Bailey, Jr. & Wolery, 1989).

The skills tested in a criterion-referenced test are generally listed in developmental sequence. This allows the test giver to determine the level at which the child is functioning and also allows for the measurement of the child's progress from one point in time to another. Consequently, criterion-referenced tests are well designed to measure small changes in a child's development and lend themselves to facilitate programming (Harbin, 1977).

Behavioral Observations

Behavioral observation is a critical diagnostic skill and it is imperative that it be performed in as natural a context as possible. Videotape and audiotape can be used to record behavior that can be analyzed later. When assessing a child the professional must remember to establish a rapport, use a variety of toys, schedule appointments during the best time of day for the child, assess on more than one occasion, and assess in an environment that is natural and comfortable for the child. It is a good idea to observe the child interacting with caregivers as well, to determine the interactive styles of both and to extract critical elements that impact either positively or negatively communicative interactions. The observation contexts can include playing, eating, and teaching with several caregivers and in several settings such as the home, the intervention center, and the day care center. During these observations interactive elements such as physical proximity, eye gaze behavior, types of games played, types and use of toys, and types of verbalizations of parent and child are observed and analyzed. Bailey and Wolery (1984) recommend measuring specific behaviors as they occur in one of two ways: frequency counts or duration of event recordings. For example, the clinician could analyze a thirty-minute parent-child interaction in terms of number and type of communicative acts. A frequency of occurrence count could be gathered for communicative functions (regulation, calling attention to self, etc.). This information would allow the clinician to recognize the child's communicative style and pattern, and would reveal the caregiver's responsiveness to communicative acts as well.

As part of an assessment, the interview is a critical element. Background information of the developmental history of the child can be gathered and important information regarding medical history, hearing, vision, motor development, and speech language development can be ascertained. Questionnaires are also useful; they can provide information about the parents'/caregivers' perceptions of the child's abilities.

Assessment Instruments

There are several assessment instruments available for the child from birth to five years. The items listed in Table 4-3 include those scales/assessments that

Table 4-3
Child Assessment Instruments

Assessment Instrument	Description
**Test of Auditory Comprehension of Language* (Carrow-Woolfolk) Allen, TX: DLM Teaching Resources, 1985.	measures the auditory comprehension of single words, grammatical morphemes, and elaborated sentences, and can be administered to children 3 to 8.11 years.
**Expressive One-Word Picture Vocabulary Test* (Gardner) Novato, CA: Academic Therapy Publications, 1990.	measures expressive vocabulary. It is appropriate for children 2 to 11.11 years. It is available in English and Spanish.
**Receptive One-Word Picture Vocabulary Test* (Gardner) Novato, CA: Academic Therapy Publications, 1985.	measures a child's single-word receptive vocabulary. It is appropriate for children 2 to 11.11 years. It is available in English and Spanish.
**Test of Pragmatic Skills* (Shulman) Tucson, AZ: Communication Skills Builders, 1985.	measures how children use their language in various communicative contexts. It is appropriate for children 3 to 8.11 yrs.
**Test of Early Language Development*, 2nd Ed. (Hresko, Reid, & Hammell) Austin, TX: Pro-Ed, 1991.	measures the understanding and expression of grammatical forms, language content, and semantic knowledge.
Behavioral Development Profile (Donahue, Montgomery, Keiser, Roecker, & Smith) Marshalltown, IA: Marshalltown Project, 1975.	measures the development of disabled and culturally deprived children ages birth through three. The *Profile* consists of a communication scale, motor scale, and social scale.
Birth to Three Developmental Scales (Bangs & Garrett) Hingham, MA: Teaching Resources, 1979.	provides baseline data for children birth to three years. It assesses social skills, motor skills, and receptive and expressive language.
Callier-Azusa Scales (Stillman, Ed.) Dallas, TX: Callier Center for Communications Disorders, University of Texas at Dallas, 1975.	assesses motor development, perceptual development, daily living skills, language development, and socialization. This is a developmental scale designed specifically for deaf, blind, and multidisabled children.
Carolina Developmental Profile (Lillie) Winston-Salem, NC: Kaplan School Supply	assesses fine motor, gross motor, perceptual reasoning, receptive language, expressive language. This is a criterion referenced checklist of skills expected in children two to five years.
**Communicative Evaluation Chart* (Anderson, Miles, & Matheny) Cambridge, MA: Educators Publishing Service, Inc., 1963.	assesses comprehension and expression of language and motor skills. This checklist is a screening device for children birth to five years.
The Early Intervention Developmental Profile (D'Eugenio & Rogers) Ann Arbor, MI: Early Intervention Project of Handicapped Infants and Young Children, 1975.	assesses children birth to thirty-six months in the areas of language, motor development, cognitive development, and social-emotional development. It was designed for use by a multidisciplinary team consisting of psychologist or special educator, an occupational therapist, and a speech language pathologist.

*These assessment checklists/questionnaires assess only speech/ language/communication development.

Table 4-3
Continued

Assessment Instrument	Description
**Environmental Prelanguage Battery* (Horstmeir & MacDonald) Columbus, OH: Merrill, 1978.	assesses early prelinguistic communication skills such as play, gestures, imitation, following directions. It is appropriate for the child 1 to 2.6 years.
Infant-Parent Training Program (Drezek) Austin, TX: Infant-Parent Training Program, 1973.	assesses the developmental level of children birth to one year in cognition, communication, social, and gross motor and self-help skills.
Informal Teacher Assessment Instrument (Drezek) Austin, TX: Infant Parent Training Program, 1975.	includes developmental checklists, skill checklists, observations guidelines, and checklist questions to determine developmental level of a child. It is appropriate for children birth to six years.
Koontz Child Developmental Program: Training Activities for the First 48 Months (Koontz) Los Angeles: Western Psychological Services, 1974.	assesses a child's functioning level in gross motor, fine motor, social, and language skills areas for children birth to forty-eight months.
Learning Accomplishment Profile for Infants: Experimental Edition (Griffen & Sanford) Winston-Salem, NC: Kaplan School Supply Corp., 1975.	assesses gross motor, fine motor, social, self-help, cognitive, and language areas. This assessment tool is designed to identify the developmental level of functioning in children ages birth to three.
Portage Guide to Early Education, Revised Edition (Bluma, Shearer, Frohman, & Hilliard) Portage, WI: Portage Project, 1976.	to be used as an assessment instrument to identify a child's repertoire of behaviors. It can be used for children birth to six years.
**Receptive-Expressive Emergent Language Scale* (Bzach & League) Baltimore, MD: University Park Press, 1970.	based on caregiver report and yields information on receptive and expressive language.
**Rossetti Infant Toddler Language Scale* (Rossetti) East Moline, IL: Linguisystems, 1990.	measures communication and interaction skills for children birth through three years. It looks at areas such as play, interaction attachment, pragmatics, gesture, language comprehension, and expression.
**Scales of Early Communication Skills for Hearing Impaired Children* (Moog & Geers) St. Louis, MO: Central Institution for the Deaf, 1975.	designed to assess speech and language development in hearing impaired children ages two to eight years.
**Sequenced Inventory of Communicative Development-Revised* (Hedrick, Prother, & Tobin) Seattle: University of Washington Press, 1984.	assesses language skills such as sound awareness, comprehension, and verbal expression in children three months to four years.
**Goldman-Fristoe Test of Articulation* (Goldman & Fristoe) Circle Pines, MN: American Guidance Service, 1986.	measures a child's articulation of consonant sound. It is appropriate for children two years to adult.
**Khan-Lewis Phonological Analysis* (Khan & Lewis) Circle Pines, MN: American Guidance Service, 1986.	measures L. phonological development. It is used in conjunction with the *Goldman-Fristoe Test of Articulation* and is appropriate for children two and one-half to five years.

*These assessment checklists/questionnaires assess only speech/ language/communication development.

Table 4-3
Continued

Assessment Instrument	Description
**Peabody Picture Vocabulary Test-Revised* (Dunn & Dunn) Circle Pines, MN: American Guidance Service, 1981.	assesses receptive vocabulary in children ages two and one-half years to adult. It is available in English and Spanish.
**Clinical Evaluation of Language Fundamentals-P* (Wiig, Secord, & Semel) San Antonio, TX: Psychological Corporation, 1992.	measures a range of expressive and receptive language skills in preschool children ages three through six.
**Preschool Language Scale-3* (Zimmerman, Steiner, & Pond) San Antonio, TX: Psychological Corporation, 1992.	assesses auditory comprehension and verbal language for children birth to 6.11 years. It is available in English and Spanish.
Early Language Milestone (ELM) Scale-2 (Caplan) Austin, TX: Pro-Ed, 1993.	considers several communicative behaviors such as receptive, expressive, visual for children birth to 36 months.
Utah Test of Language Development-3 (Mecham & Jones) Austin, TX: Pro-Ed, 1989.	assesses the expressive and receptive language of children three through nine.

*These assessment checklists/questionnaires assess only speech/language/communication development.

test across multiple domains such as motor development, language development, cognitive development, and social emotional development.

Assessment Areas

The areas that must be considered when assessing the infant/toddler/preschool child include cognitive development, communicative development, development of play, and motor development.

Cognitive Development

Piaget (1952) developed a model of the development of cognition that extends from birth to fourteen years. This model is particularly interesting to educators in planning intervention techniques (see Table 4-4). Also of interest and use to the assessment team are scales that assess the earliest cognitive development. Several such scales have been developed that utilize this Piagetian framework; Uzgiris and Hunt (1975) have developed six scales that pertain to the six branches of psychological development of infants.

An offshoot of Piagetian theory of cognitive development that is useful in assessing young children is information processing theory, which considers the mind as a complex cognitive system (Paget, 1989). This complex system is regarded in terms of mental processes that enable the child to problem solve and process cognition.

Table 4-4
Piagetian Stages of Cognitive Development

Stage		Chronological Age
Stage I	Sensorimotor Period	Birth to 24 months
Stage II	Prioperational Period	2 to 7 years
Stage III	Concrete Operation Period	7 to 11 years
Stage IV	Formal Operations Period	11 to 14 years

Play Development

Play is the child's domain. Assessment of play will give the evaluation team valuable information about how a child interacts with his or her environment. Westby (1980) developed a scale that describes symbolic play and integrates expected language structures with play performance. Garvey (1974) developed a scale of play stages that integrates Piaget's stages of cognitive development with play. Another play assessment instrument that looks at social play is Howes's Peer Play Scale (1980), which considers five developmental levels of play and allows the examiner to determine at what level the child is functioning based on observations of play.

Besides being an enjoyable activity, play serves as a vehicle to practice and solidify cognitive skills, promote emotional and social growth, refine gross and fine motor skills, and enhance communication development (Wolery & Bailey, Jr., 1989). As the child grows older it is expected that play schemas become more elaborate, complex, and interactive. When a child's level of play is assessed and understood, it is a valuable resource for facilitating development of other behaviors.

Motor Development

Normal motor development is well documented (Chandler, 1979; Knoblock & Passamanick, 1974); children pass through motor developmental milestones in an orderly fashion. Consequently, assessment of motor development is easily managed and is typically divided into assessment of fine motor skills and gross motor skills. The areas that should be considered when conducting a motor assessment include muscle tone, reflexes and reaction, movement and posture patterns, and functional abilities (Smith, 1989).

Recently much research has centered on the development of oral motor skills in the infant. Oral motor functioning includes reflexive oral motor abilities such as sucking and swallowing; assessment of feeding is especially important when working with the child who has suspected motor disabilities. In addition, study of the early vocal behaviors of the infant is of particular interest to the SLP. The chronology of oral motor feeding patterns is as follows.

Birth to Six Months

Suckling: extension-retraction of tongue, up-and-down jaw movement, loose lip approximation.

Sucking: rhythmic up-and-down jaw movements with tongue tip elevation, tight approximation of the lips.

Rooting: head turns in response to tactile stimulation of lips or mouth.

Phasic bite reflex: rhythmic bite and release pattern when gums are stimulated.

Six to Twenty-Four Months

Munching: earliest level of chewing in which the tongue is flat and the jaw moves up and down.

Chewing: food is propelled between the teeth through spreading and rolling movements of tongue.

Tongue lateralization: the tongue moves to the sides of the mouth and propels food between teeth for chewing.

Rotary jaw movements: integration of vertical, lateral, diagonal, and circular movements of the jaw during chewing.

Controlled bite: easy closure of teeth on food with easy releasing of food for chewing (Jaffe, 1989).

Formal feeding assessment instruments include *The Feeding Assessment*, in English and Spanish versions (Morris & Klein, 1987); *The Pre-Speech Assessment Scale* (Morris, 1982); and *Oral Motor Assessment* (Sleight & Niman, 1984). Each of these instruments will enable the SLP to identify any strengths or needs associated with feeding.

The normally developing infant learns to shape vocalizations into sound productions that approximate words and, eventually, multiword productions. For the infant with oral motor difficulties the process does not necessarily occur with ease. Although there are no norms for articulatory and acoustic data on non-cry vocal behaviors in infancy, there are available research studies that examine infant vocalizations (Oller, 1980, 1986; Delack & Fowlow, 1978). Proctor (1989) delineates five stages of vocal development and has developed a vocal assessment form.

Stage 1: There are more crying sounds than non-crying sounds; non-crying sounds are mostly vegetative.

Stage 2: Less crying; predominance of vocalic sounds, LV productions.

Stage 3: Increased consonant productions; varied vowel productions; consistent CV syllables; varied intonation contours.

Stage 4: Reduplicated babbling in the form of CV or CVC structures; consistent variations in intonation contours.

Stage 5: Variety of CV and CVC combinations with sentencelike intonation; approximations of meaningful single words.

Utilization of a protocol such as Proctor's enables the SLP to determine level of vocal behavior development, compare it with oral motor feeding skill level development, and plan therapeutic intervention.

Stoel-Gammon (1987) states that by two years of age the normally developing child produces words using CV, CVC, CVCV, and CVCVC form; produces a few consonant clusters; matches the consonant phonemes of adult words with 70 percent correctness; produces nine or ten different consonants in initial position; and produces five or six different consonants in the final position. This information is also useful to the SLP in determining whether intervention is needed for the young preschool child.

CULTURAL DIFFERENCES

The early intervention professional working with disabled infants and toddlers must be keenly aware that just as all special-needs children are not alike, the families of all special-needs children are not alike. Families differ in terms of cultural backgrounds, economic conditions, and family structure. Bailey (1987) cautions that it is not inconceivable that the professional will be faced with values that conflict with his or her own values. These differences in values may be due to culture, religious background, or socioeconomic status; sometimes they are due to the parents' acceptance of the child's disabling condition or the professional's philosophical orientation. Aponte (1985) cautions the professional to understand family structures, family values, and family functions.

Family Standards and Values

Family values are standards; families make decisions based on those standards. Family structure is the organizational framework of the family, i.e., the individual roles of family members. Family functioning is the way the family works to achieve or accomplish goals. The professional must identify those areas of functioning that need support or help. There are several scales that determine those needs areas. The *Coping—Health Inventory for Parents* (McCubbin, McCubbin, Nevin, & Cauble, 1979), which was designed for families with special-needs children, identifies the family's perceptions regarding the management needs of the disabled child. The *Family Roles Scale* (Gallagher, Scharfman, & Bristol, 1984), a measure of role performance in the family, identifies who is currently responsible for most child care and is most helpful when considering intervention strategies and IFSP goals. Another measure of family functioning, the *Family Adjustment Survey* (Abbott & Meredith,

1986), determines a family's coping style, its strengths, and its support systems. All of these scales provide insights into the unique style and structure of special-needs families. It is also important to determine what the family itself considers of primary importance in terms of needs. Bailey, Jr. and Simeonsson (1988) highlight several needs areas of parents, such as the need for information, for family support, for help in explaining their child's problem to others, for help in getting community services, and financial and intrafamily functioning needs.

In addition, professionals must be aware of the cultural history and traditions of families. Anderson (1992) highlights the fact that culturally different families may have different expectations and aspirations for their children. She emphasizes that professionals need to listen to families in order to recognize and appreciate these differences. Most assessment instruments have been normed on white middle-class populations. Even though there have been attempts to establish culturally adjusted tests, these attempts have not been completely successful.

Difference vs. Disorder

Children of different cultures may develop at different rates. Cultural differences do not constitute disorders. For example, Western cultures place high priorities on language development, while many foreign cultures place priorities on silence. With these differences in mind the professional team must assess with an unbiased perspective.

During the last three decades educators have been struggling with societal issues of difference versus disorder and monocultural versus pluralistic ideology. The fields of special education and bilingual education developed separately; children who were culturally and linguistically different were often considered disabled. When bilingual education programs grew, another equally disturbing outcome occurred. Many minority children with disabling conditions were not identified as such, but were placed in bilingual classrooms without the necessary services their conditions necessitated (Omark & Erickson, 1983). Fortunately we have learned from our mistakes and recognize the need to discriminate between cultural differences and actual language disorders.

By the year 2000 it is expected that over three million children of non–English-speaking backgrounds will be living in the United States. We must be prepared to identify exceptional children in their linguistic and cultural milieu (Bergin, 1980). This is no easy task. The clinician must be sensitive to the cultural characteristics of a child's ethnic community; he or she must also be knowledgeable regarding acquisition and normative data on the child's first language.

The 1990 U.S. census revealed that one-fourth of the people in the United States are nonwhite. Twelve percent are African-American, 9 percent are Hispanic, 3 percent are Asian/Pacific American, and 1 percent Native American and Eskimo (Taylor, 1993). Speech/language clinicians need to have sufficient knowledge regarding diverse cultural groups in order to provide competent clinical services to these children and their families. Cultural groups have unique cultural characteristics; understanding of salient cultural and linguistic factors is necessary for assessment and treatment of communication disorders.

African Americans are the largest minority population in the United States. A large proportion of this highly diverse group are descendants of forced emigration to this country with subsequent economic and political enslavement (Terrel & Terrel, 1993). Let us consider the following useful information from Terrel and Terrel regarding the assessment of African-American children. An important cultural value of this community revolves around names and titles. Today many African-American children have names with unusual pronunciations or spellings that may be African names. It may be insulting to the family if a clinician uses a diminutive of the name. A good rule is to ask the family the name preference. Clinicians should also always address parents with their formal titles—Mr., Mrs., Doctor, or Ms., for example. Do not make the mistake of calling a parent by his or her first name in an effort to create informality and friendliness.

Several linguistic dialects are spoken among African Americans. The most predominant is Black English; however, others include Gullah (used by people living on islands near the coast of South Carolina and Georgia), Jamaica Creole, English, and dialects spoken by people from the Caribbean or African nations.

Black English is an American English dialect and consists of rule-governed, grammatical, phonological, syntactic, semantic, and pragmatic features. Not all African Americans speak Black English, and the factors that influence its degree of usage include age, geographic location, income, occupation, and education (Labov, 1966). Phonological rules include: 1. silencing or substituting the consonants in a word (*day* for *they, brovah* for *brother*); 2. silencing unstressed initial phonemes and unstressed initial syllables (*bout* for *about*); 3. silencing the final consonant in a consonant cluster (*mas* for *mask*). Morphological and syntactical differences are extensive and beyond the scope of this chapter. Cole (1980), Dillard (1973), Labov (1966), and Taylor (1986) provide in-depth treatment of this subject. However, the clinician working with African-American children should note that Cole (1980) documented normal acquisition of Black English patterns and suggests that because of the difference in developmental patterns it is difficult to identify language disorders utilizing conventional language tests.

Eye contact, narrative style, and code switching are additional cultural differences that must be recognized as such and not considered disordered. For example, some African-American children do not establish eye contact with an adult during a conversation because to do so would be disrespectful. Furthermore, children proficient only in Black English will use fewer words and less elaboration in school situations. However, in more familiar, informal settings these children are more talkative and elaborate. Terrel and Terrel (1993) have also identified a narrative style difference among Black English children. Rather than adhering to a central topic during a discussion, African-American children may utilize an associational discussion style. For instance, when a child is asked to talk about what he or she saw and did at the circus, mainstream expectation would be for the child to talk only about things seen or done at the circus. However, the African-American child may make a statement that is generated from what another child said previously about the circus. An example of this style would be as follows: First child states that she saw a clown at the circus; the second child says that he saw clowns on TV; the third child adds that he likes to watch cartoons on TV. This type of discussion narrative should not be considered off-topic or tangential, but rather a culturally different style of narration.

Asian-Pacific Americans are a diverse group of people who have various ethnic backgrounds and include Chinese, Japanese, Indochinese, Pacific Islanders, Koreans, and Filipinos. Each cultural group has its own set of values, norms, beliefs, attitudes, and behavioral styles. Cheng (1993) discusses these groups; the following is a summary of her findings.

In China there are over eighty languages and several hundred dialects in use. These languages are noninflectional; in Mandarin Chinese only two final consonants—*n* and *y*—are present, and in Cantonese only seven. Consequently, Chinese speakers will frequently omit final consonants when speaking English. The pragmatic rules of the Chinese language are also quite different from those of English and it is not uncommon for a woman to break eye contact with a speaker and gaze down.

The Japanese language is polysyllabic and has an elaborate inflectional system. There are five vowels and eighteen consonants and only the *n* phoneme is used in the final position of words.

The Korean language utilizes no word stress and there are no labiodental, interdental, or palatal fricatives in the language. Pragmatically, silence is an important part of communication.

The various other languages of Asian-American peoples utilize individual phonetic, semantic, syntactic, and pragmatic rules that differ from those of English. Because traditional assessment approaches may not effectively measure communicative competence, the clinician must rethink the assessment process. Cheng (1993) suggests a communication assessment that considers the child in his or her unique cultural and linguistic environment. This ethnographic assessment includes naturalistic contexts and behavioral descriptions. The clinician must address the following:

1. What are the child's purposes for communicating?
2. When does the child's communication break down?
3. How does the child communicate with family members?
4. Is the child successful in communicating wants and needs?
5. What does the child communicate?
6. Are there other important environmental factors that should be considered?

Hispanic persons have different cultural backgrounds, socioeconomic levels, and educational levels. The Hispanic population in the United States comprises 9 percent of the total population and includes Mexican Americans, Puerto Ricans, Central and South Americans, and Cubans (Kayser, 1993). Because of the large numbers of Hispanic persons in the United States and the continuous arrival of new immigrants who maintain the minority language, Hispanic children often need to develop two languages. The Hispanic population is heterogeneous and varies in the ways they socialize and interact with their children. Although Spanish and English share many phonemes, there is not a one-to-one correspondence, and they differ in their phonological rules. For instance, final clusters do not occur in Spanish and *s* blends do not occur in the initial position. Kayser (1993) has delineated the morphosyntactic and semantic development of Spanish-speaking children. She states that these children use single words before two years of age, two-word constructions by age two, and three-word constructions by age three. By age four and a half, the child is using thirty-eight Spanish syntactic structures (Garcia & Gonzales, 1984). An assessment of a bilingual Hispanic child should always include the status of both languages in the child's environment and consideration of the linguistic and cultural variables in that environment.

In general, an ethnographic approach is imperative in providing speech language services to culturally diverse groups. We need to directly observe the child interacting with caregivers in a familiar environment. Slobin (1967) states that we should observe the child and the family over time in order to gather data regarding caregiving style, attitude toward communicative skills, importance of eye contact, and the family's communicative pattern.

When using standardized measures it is important to determine who the subjects in the sampling data were. Generally, ethnic minority groups are not included and the test data must be interpreted cautiously, understanding that cultural biases exist.

Use of nonstandardized procedures such as gathering and analyzing a conversational sample is highly useful. Use culturally familiar objects/toys to encourage verbalizations and, when analyzing this sample, compare the child's performance in light of the language variables of his or her culture. Terrel, Arensberg, and Rosa (1992) developed a *Parent Child Comparative Analysis* (PCCA) that can be used to compare the child's communicative patterns to that of the family. When the child's pattern does not match that of the caregiver and does not meet the expectations for the child's chronological age, there is a possibility of a language disorder.

Determining whether a communication disorder exists in a culturally different child requires a clear determination of whether the apparent communication difficulty is a product of language difference or language disorder. The clinician must utilize modified test procedures, adapt existing tests, and gather a language sample that reflects the child's naturalistic communication pattern (Kayser, 1993). Some of these test modifications may include omitting items that you expect the child to miss because of language or culture, continuing testing beyond the ceiling, and rewarding instructions. Taylor

(1986) explains these modifications in detail. In some instances, especially when standardized tests are administered, an interpreter must be used. Bernstein (1989) cautions that the interpreter must be involved with the assessment team throughout the assessment process and should have the freedom to ask questions.

In summary, when assessing the preschool child the task is to assess *communicative competence,* which is determined by the norms of the child's community of speakers. We must understand that the communicative norms of a mainstream society are not necessarily the communicative norms for the minority child that we are evaluating. A good rule of thumb is to gather a detailed family case history and identify the parents' concerns regarding the child's communication. Observe the child in various settings and use questionnaires and interviews to assist in the identification process. Take into consideration how cultural differences affect testing, and expand your knowledge of the cultural group you are testing. One must observe and describe the child's communicative pattern in a naturalistic setting and not consider the mainstream norm as the sole standard for comparison and determination of disorder. Hansen, Lynch, and Wayman (1990) offer the following suggestions for professionals when gathering ethnographic information.

1. When working with a child from a different culture, describe the ethnic group in terms of the family's country of origin, language, and number of people in the ethnic community.
2. Be aware of the social organization of the ethnic community and resources in that community.
3. Be aware of the belief system in the community, such as ceremonies, values, and symbols.
4. Be aware of the current events in the ethnic community that impact the family directly.
5. Be aware of the attitudes in the ethnic community toward seeking help.

In evaluating the culturally different child the evaluator must utilize a pluralistic assessment approach. This approach might include using criterion-referenced measures (Mowder, 1980) or developing locally normed measures (Watson, Omark, Grouell, & Heller, 1980). Criterion-referenced assessments consist of determining what behaviors are expected for a particular age range and then observing those behaviors in the child being assessed.

Developing locally normed measures would solve the problem of valid assessment for culturally different children. However, most educators do not have expertise in test development and construction nor do they have the time to dedicate to such a task. Toronto and Merrill (1983) caution that although the locally normed instrument is a valuable tool it should never be used as a sole determinant of diagnosis or placement.

Ecological Validity

Ecological validity is another important issue when working with culturally different children and families. We must ensure that our assessment instruments have ecological validity and that they are sensitive to cultural differences and do not penalize a child for these differences. Culture and language are factors in national identity. If we want to understand people we must understand their culture; if we want to assess children we must understand their culture.

A useful assessment technique that facilitates ecological validity is naturalistic observation. This evaluation approach involves the recording of ongoing behavior without attempting to influence it (McBurney, 1991). Careful record keeping is of paramount importance. The evaluator keeps a record of the behavior of interest and under what circumstances it occurs. By using movie cameras and videotape recorders with slow-motion options and stop-action freeze, the evaluator is able to recognize critical behavior patterns. The evaluation should focus on specific types of social, communicative, and cognitive behaviors. Note what language is used by the caregiver and in what language the child responds (Linares, 1983). There may be instances in which the evaluator wishes to join the caregiver and the child and conduct a participant-observer observation. When this occurs, it is important to continue to videotape the interactions and determine what changes occur. Later analysis of the videotapes will give the evaluator insights into the cultural social rules of the family.

Another useful assessment tool is the language sample, which provides an in-depth description of a child's communication skills in a natural setting. If the language sample is collected appropriately, the educator can get a good understanding of the child's production abilities. It is not within the scope of this chapter to train the professional to gather and analyze a language sample. However, when utilizing this assessment procedure the clinician must consider six variables: nature of the interaction, setting, materials, sample size, method of recording, and specification of context (Stickler, 1987). Nature of the interaction refers to the person with whom the child is interacting and whether or not that person asks questions or generally converses during interactive play. Setting refers to the actual environment in which the sample is gathered. Miller (1981) recommended several alternatives to the therapy room, such as the home or the classroom. Materials are another important variable. Miller reported that new and unique toys generate more language from language-disordered children. Nisswandt (1983), on the other hand, reported the opposite effect of using new and unique toys with language-normal children. That is, these materials generated less spontaneous language production. Sample size refers to the number of utterances gathered. Some investigators recommend a language sample of at least 100 communicative acts (Tyack & Gottsleben, 1975) while others recommend between 200 and 300 (Muma, 1978). This clinician feels that with a very young child (one to three years) a sample of 100 utterances is sufficient, while with an older child (three to five years) a 200-utterance sample is more representative. There are three methods of recording: videotaping, audiotaping, and on-line transcription. The most preferred method is videotaping; it allows for complete delineation of both verbal and nonverbal contexts. However, when used correctly the other two methods can also provide reliable valid measures of spontaneous speech production. Specification of context refers to the utterances of the other conversational participants in the language sample setting as well as notation of the nonverbal or situational context. This variable is quite important to the interpretation of the child's utterances.

Once a child is identified as having a disability, variables such as age of the child, attitudes and goals of the family, potential for communication skills, and available social interactions must all be considered when developing an educational plan. It cannot be automatically assumed that the disabled minority child should receive intervention in English. As a pluralistic society we must break away from our monocultural perspective and recognize that there must be an integration and match between a child's culture and that of the educational system. When working with the culturally different child whose first language is not English, the early educator needs to recognize that emphasis should be placed on native language development, because strong development of the native language will foster a good acquisition of the second language (English).

When minority speech and hearing professionals are not available to evaluate a culturally different child, it is necessary to utilize paraprofessionals in the identification and intervention process. In 1970 ASHA published *Guidelines for Supportive Personnel in Speech Pathology and Audiology.* It was recognized that these paraprofessionals can assist and enhance the effectiveness of the speech language intervention with the culturally different child. They can assist the educator in recording, translating, and analyzing spontaneous speech samples; they can sensitize the educator to cultural customs and social rules; they help the educator understand the disorders of non–English- or limited–English-speaking children.

THE AT-RISK CHILD

The term *at-risk* means different things to different professionals. The physician considers the at-risk child as one who has a fragile medical condition that impacts negatively physical growth and development. The speech pathologist considers the at-risk child as one who has experienced or is experiencing circumstances that impact negatively speech and language development and later academic performance. Some of the environmental conditions that put a child at risk are prematurely low birth weight, familial history of speech delay, difficult birth (such as prolonged labor), serious injury, or illness. Any extraordinary factor during prenatal or postnatal periods puts an infant at risk for developmental delay. According to Rossetti (1989) approximately 5 to 15 percent of all live-born infants can be considered at-risk infants and 55,000 infants per year are identified as disabled. These infants experience an increased susceptibility to developmental delay, educational delays, poor peer relationships, abuse, and neglect.

There have been a number of follow-up studies on the high-risk population (Babson, 1970; Rubin, Rosenblatt, & Balow, 1973; Maisels & Marks, 1981; Rosen, 1982). The studies that are particularly interesting to the SLP examine the speech development of these children. In particular, studies that focus on very low birth weight (VLBW) infants have shown that the incidence of hearing loss among these children is fourteen times greater than in the general population (Downs, 1982). In addition, although these VLBW infants do develop non-vocal communication early, their expressive speech is delayed, with only a few words exhibited at the age of eighteen to twenty-four months (Rossetti, 1989). Other researchers (Hubatch, Johnson, Kistler, Bruns, & Moneka, 1985) compared the receptive and expressive language skills of VLBW children and normal birth weight children at eighteen to twenty months. Their results indicated that the VLBW children had significantly less receptive and expressive skills than their normal birth weight peers. Studies that focused on later school performance of VLBW infants show that these children experience academic delays. Francis-Williams and Davies (1974) looked at the reading levels of these children; 30 percent displayed problems in learning to read. Drillen, Thomson, and Burgoyne (1980) examined differences between low birth weight (LBW) children and their peers at age six to seven on measures of reading ability, visuomotor ability, and speech and language skills; they found the LBW children's performance significantly poorer. Steiner, Sanders, Phillips, and Maddock (1980) looked at reading performance of VLBW children and their normal birth weight peers and found that reading performance of more than 50 percent of the VLBW children was two or more years below average.

SUMMARY

Inherent in the term *early intervention* are concepts such as flexibility, sensitivity, respect, collaboration, nontraditional, and creativity. Inherent in the term *early childhood service providers* are concepts such as listener, teacher, partner, and friend. In order to meet the challenge of early intervention we must revolutionize our thinking. We are no longer simply the teachers of children or diagnosticians. We are partners in a collaborative relationship that is based on trust and respect. Yes, we still diagnose, we still teach. But just as Public Law 99-457 expanded the boundaries of special education, so too does it expand our professional horizons. We must expand our way of thinking about who we are and what we do.

We no longer provide services only to the child. Instead we work with the family and the child in order to facilitate development in multiple areas such as communication, play, and social interaction. Our relationship is a collaborative one. We model strategies for the parent and the parent interacts with the child.

We provide direct intervention to the child and to the family. We identify family strengths and needs and child strengths and needs. We work through the strengths to diminish the needs.

We utilize a variety of standardized assessment instruments to determine how a child performs in relation to his or her peers. We use observations, questionnaires, interviews, and home visits to determine how the child functions in the home environment and what the expectations are for this child in this environment.

We generate our goals based on the data gathered from the family, from our own observations and testing, and from the testing and observations of other professionals. These goals are a collaborative effort. They reflect goals that cross disciplines and meet family and child needs.

Public Law 99-457 has challenged us. It has dared us to look into our therapy mirrors, our looking glass, and to go beyond what was—and to enter into what can be.

A FEW WORDS FROM TOYA DAVIS

I knew very early on that my son Jonathan had a problem. My journey began when I had the courage to pursue my gut feeling and seek out professionals who confirmed my uneasiness about Jonathan's speech language development. Once his problem was identified I had to embark on a personal journey of grieving over the "death" of my idealized perfect child, Jonathan. I had to embrace the real Jonathan, the Jonathan who was still the love of my life, but was somewhat less than perfect. With all that in mind I want to emphasize how important the communication was between the professionals who worked with Jonathan and me. It was important that I had access to them, that I could speak to them and they could hear what I said. In order for the professional to hear me, to hear my concerns, to understand me, to assess Jonathan, he/she had to recognize that Jonathan existed in our family, which existed in our extended family, which existed in our cultural community. Our heritage consists of customs, values, beliefs, behaviors that give us our identities. Our spoken language is enriched with dialectical variations. Our family customs were different from those of the evaluators and there had to be an understanding and respect for that. However, Jonathan still needed intervention and I looked to the professional to evaluate his strengths and needs with an understanding of differences not necessarily implying disorder. In retrospect I realize that what I want for me, for Jonathan, for all families who enter into the special education process is that their heritage, their culture, their values are recognized, appreciated, and respected. It is only through mutual respect and understanding that valid assessments of family needs and child needs can be ascertained. It is only through mutual respect and understanding that trust can develop between the professionals and the families they serve.

REFERENCES

Abbott, D. A., & Meredith, W. H. (1986). Strengths of parents with retarded children. *Family Relations, 35,* 371–375.

American Speech Language Hearing Association (1990). The roles of speech-language pathologists in service delivery to infants, toddlers, and their families. *ASHA, 32* (Suppl. 2), 4.

Anderson, N. B. (1992). Changes in cultural demographics warrant shift in approach to diagnosis, treatment. *Advance, 2,* 5.

Aponte, H. J. (1985). The negotiation of values in therapy. *Family Process, 24,* 323–338.

Babson, S. (1970). Growth of low birthweight infants. *Journal of Pediatrics, 77,* 11.

Bailey, D. (1991). Preparing professionals to serve infants and toddlers with handicaps and their families: An integrative analyses across eight disciplines. *Exceptional Children, 57* (1), 26–35.

Bailey, D. B. (1987). Collaboration goal setting with families: Resolving differences in values and priorities for services. *Topics in Early Childhood Special Education, 7* (2), 59–71.

Bailey, D. B., & Wolery, M. (1984). *Teaching infants and preschoolers with handicaps.* New York: Merrill/Macmillan.

Bailey, D., Jr., & Simeonsson, R. (1988). *Family assessment in early intervention.* New York: Merrill/Macmillan.

Bailey, D., Jr., & Wolery, M. (1989). *Assessing infants and preschoolers with handicaps.* New York: Merrill/Macmillan.

Bell, R. Q. (1968). A reinterpretation of the direction of effects in studies of socialization. *Psychological Review, 75,* 81–95.

Bell, R. Q., & Harper, L. V. (1977). *Child effects on adults.* Hillsdale, NJ: Lawrence Erlbaum.

Bergin, V. (1980). *Special education needs in bilingual programs.* Washington, DC: National Clearinghouse for Bilingual Education.

Bernstein, D. (1989). Assessing children with limited English proficiency: Current perspectives. *Topics in Language Disorders, 9* (3), 15–20.

Brazelton, T. B. (1982). Joint regulation of neonati-parent behavior. In E. Z. Tronick (Ed.), *Social interchange in infancy: Affect, cognition, and communication* (pp. 7–22). Baltimore: University Park Press.

Bronfenbrenner, U. (1977). Toward an experimental ecology of human development. *American Psychologist, 32,* 513–531.

Chandler, L. (1979). Gross and fine motor development. In M. Cohen & P. Gross (Eds.), *The developmental resource: Behavioral sequences for assessment and program planning* (Vol. 1) (pp 119–152). New York: Grune & Stratton.

Cheng, L. L. (1993). Asian American cultures. In D. Battle (Ed.), *Communication disorders in multicultural populations* (pp. 38–77). Boston: Andover Medical Publications.

Cole, L. (1980). *Developmental analysis of social dialect features in the sponta-*

neous language of preschool black children. Evanston, IL: Northwestern University (thesis).

Crais, E., & Roberts, J. (1991). Decision making in assessment and early intervention planning. *Language, Speech, and Hearing Services in Schools, 22,* 19–30.

Delack, J. B. (1976). Aspects of infant speech development in the first year of life. *Canadian Journal of Linguistics, 21,* 17–37.

Delack, J. B., & Fowlow, P. J. (1978). The ontogenesis of differential vocalization: Development of prosodic contrastivity during the first year of life. In N. Waterson & C. Snow (Eds.), *The development of communication.* New York: Wiley & Sons.

Dillard, J. L. (1973). *Black English: Its history and usage in the United States.* New York: Vintage Books.

Downs, M. (1982). Early identification of hearing loss. In M. Lass, J. N. McReynolds, & D. Yoder (Eds.), *Speech, language and hearing* (Vol. III, Hearing disorders). Philadelphia: W. B. Saunders.

Drillen, C., Thomson, A., & Burgoyne, K. (1980). Low birth weight children at early school age: A longitudinal study. *Developmental Medicine and Child Neurology, 22,* 26.

Dunst, C., & Trivette, C. (1988). *Enabling and empowering families: Principles and guidelines for practice.* Cambridge, MA: Brookline Books.

Family support in the home: Home visiting program and PL 99-457. (1988). Washington, DC: Association for the Care of Children's Health.

Farran, N. C., Kasari, C., Yoder, P., Harber, L., Huntington, O. S., & Comfort-Smith, M. (1987). Rating mother child interactions in handicapped and at-risk infants. In T. Tamer (Ed.), *Stimulation intervention in infant development.* London: Freund Publishing House.

Francis-Williams, J., & Davies, P. (1974). Very low birth weight and later intelligence. *Developmental Medicine and Child Neurology, 16,* 709.

Gallagher, J. J., Scharfman, W., & Bristol, M. (1984). The division of responsibilities in families with preschool handicapped and nonhandicapped children. *Journal of the Division for Early Childhood, 8,* 3–12.

Garcia, E., & Gonzalez, G. (1984). The interrelationship of Spanish and Spanish/English language acquisition in the Hispanic child. In J. V. Martinez & R. H. Mendoza (Eds.), *Chicano psychology,* 2nd ed. New York: Academic Press.

Garvey, C. (1974). Some properties of social play. *Merrill Palmer Quarterly, 20,* 163–180.

Harbin, G. (1977). Educational assessment. In L. Cross & K. Goin (Eds.), *Identifying handicapped children* (pp. 35–52). Chapel Hill: University of North Carolina.

Hansen, M., Lynch, E., & Wayman, K. (1990). Honoring the cultural diversity of families when gathering data. *Topics in Language Disorders, 10* (1), 112–131.

Howes, C. (1980). Peer play scale as an index of complexity of peer interaction. *Developmental Psychology, 16,* 371–372

Hubatch, L., Johnson, C., Kistler, D., Bruns, W., & Moneka, W. (1985). Early language abilities of high risk infants. *Journal of Speech and Hearing Disorders, 5,* 195.

Jaffe, M. (1989). Feeding at-risk infants and toddlers. *Topics in Language Disorders, 10* (1), 13–25.

Kayser, H. (1993). Hispanic cultures. In D. Battle (Ed.), *Communication disorders in multicultural populations* (pp. 114–57). Boston: Andover Medical Publications.

Knoblock, H., & Passamanick, B. (1974). *Gesell and Amatruda's developmental diagnoses: The evaluation and management of normal and neuropsychologic development in infancy and early childhood.* New York: Harper & Row.

Labov, W. (1966). *The social stratifications of English in New York City.* Washington, DC: Center for Applied Linguistics.

Lewis, M., & Rosenblum, J. (Eds.) (1974). *The effects of the infant on its caregiver.* New York: John Wiley and Sons.

Linares, N. (1983). Management of communicatively handicapped Hispanic children. In D. R. Omark & J. G. Erickson (Eds.), *The bilingual exceptional child.* Boston: College-Hill Press.

Maisels, J., & Marks, K. (1981). Growth chart for sick premature infants. *Journal of Pediatrics, 98,* 66.

McBurney, D. (1991). *Experimental psychology* (2nd ed.). Belmont, CA: Wadsworth Publishing Co.

McCollum, J. (1984). Social interaction between parents and babies: Validation of an intervention procedure. *Child: Care, Health and Development, 10,* 301–315.

McCollum, J., & Hughes, M. (1988). Staffing patterns and team models in infancy programs. In J. Jordan, J. Gallagher, P. Hutinger, and M. Karnes (Eds.), *Early childhood special education: Birth to three* (pp. 129–146). Reston, VA: The Council for Exceptional Children.

McCollum, J., & Stayton, V. D. (1985). Infant/parent interaction: Studies and intervention guidelines based on the SIAI model. *Journal of the Division for Early Childhood, 9* (2), 125–135.

McCubbin, H. I., McCubbin, M., Nevin, R., & Cauble, E. (1979). *Coping—Help Inventory For Parents.* Unpublished rating scales, School of Family and Social Sciences, University of Minnesota–St. Paul.

Miller, J. (1981). *Assessing language production in children: Experimental procedures.* Baltimore: University Park Press.

Morris, S. E. (1982). *Pre-speech assessment scale.* Clifton, NJ: J. A. Preston.

Morris, S. E., & Klein, M. D. (1987). *Pre-feeding skills.* Tucson, AZ: Therapy Skill Builders.

Mowder, B. A. (1980). A strategy for the assessment of bilingual handicapped children. *Psychology in the Schools, 17,* 7–11.

Muma, J. R. (1978). *Language handbook.* Englewood Cliffs, NJ: Prentice-Hall.

Nisswandt, B. (1983). *The effects of situational variability on the grammatical speech forms of three-year-olds.* Unpublished master's thesis, University of Wisconsin, Eau Claire.

Oller, D. K. (1980). The emergence of the sounds of speech in infancy. In G. A. Yeri-Komshian, J. F. Kavanagh, & C. A. Ferguson (Eds.), *Child phonology* (Vol. 1: Production). New York: Academic Press.

Oller, D. K. (1986). Metaphonology and infant vocalization. In B. Lindblom & R. Zetterstrom (Eds.), *Precursors of early speech* (pp. 21–35). New York: Stockton Press.

Omark, D. R., & Erickson, J. G. (Eds.). (1983). *The bilingual exceptional child.* Boston: College-Hill Press.

Paget, K. (1989). Assessment of cognitive skills in the preschool aged child. In D. Bailey, Jr. & M. Wolery (Eds.), *Assessing infants and preschoolers with handicaps* (pp. 275–300). New York: Merrill/Macmillan.

Piaget J. (1952). *The origins of intelligence in children.* New York: International Universities Press.

Proctor, A. (1989). Stages of normal noncry vocal development in infancy: A protocol for assessment. *Topics in Language Disorders, 10* (1), 26–42.

Rosen, M. (1982). The biological vulnerability of a low birth weight infant. In D. Parron & L. Eisenberg (Eds.), *Infants at risk for developmental dysfunction.* (Health and Behavior: A Research Agenda: Interim Rep. No. 4). Washington, DC: National Academy Press.

Rosenberg, S., Robinson, C., & Beckman, P. (1984). Teaching skills inventory: A measure of parent performance. *Journal of the Division for Early Childhood, 8,* 107–113.

Rossetti, L. (1989). *High-risk infants: Identification, assessment, and intervention.* Boston: College-Hill Press.

Rubin, R., Rosenblatt, C., & Balow, B. (1973). Psychological and educational sequelae of prematurity. *Pediatrics, 52,* 352.

Sleight, M., & Niman, C. (1984). *Gross motor and oral motor development in children with Down Syndrome: Birth through three years.* St. Louis: St. Louis Association for Retarded Citizens.

Slobin, D. I. (Ed.) (1967). *A field manual for cross-cultural study of the acquisition of communicative competence.* Berkeley, CA: University of California.

Smith, P. (1989). Assessing motor skills. In D. Bailey, Jr. & M. Wolery (Eds.), *Assessing Infant and Preschoolers with Handicaps* (pp. 301–338). New York: Merrill/Macmillan.

Soper, E. H. (1991). Reflections on Part H: One state's experience. *Infants and Young Children, 4* (1), I–VIII.

Steiner, F., Sanders, E., Phillips, E., & Maddock, C. (1980). Very low birth weight children at school age: Comparison of neonatal management methods. *British Medical Journal, 281,* 1237.

Stickler, K. R. (1987). *Guide to analysis of language transcripts.* Eau Claire, WI: Thinking Publications.

Stoel-Gammon, C. (1987). Phonological skills of 2-year-olds. *Language, Speech, and Hearing Services in Schools, 18,* 323–329.

Taylor, O. (Ed.). (1986). *Nature of communication disorders in culturally and linguistically diverse populations.* San Diego, CA: College-Hill Press.

Taylor, O. (1993). Foreword. In D. Battle (Ed.), *Communication disorders in multicultural populations* (p. 11). Boston: Andover Medical Publishers.

Terrel, S., & Terrel, F. (1993). African American cultures. In D. Battle (Ed.), *Communication Disorders in Multicultural Populations* (pp. 3–37). Boston: Andover Medical Publications.

Terrel, S. L., Arensberg, K., & Rosa, M. (1992). Parent-child comparative analysis: A criterion-referenced method for the nondiscriminatory assessment of a child who spoke a relatively uncommon dialect of English. *Language Speech Hearing Services in the Schools, 23,* 34–42.

Thomas, A., & Chess, S. (1977). *Temperament and development.* New York: Brunner/Mazel.

Toronto, A., & Merrill, S. M. (1983). Developing local normed assessment instruments. In D. Omark & J. Erickson (Eds.), *The bilingual exceptional child* (pp. 105–121). Boston: College-Hill Press.

Tronick, E. Z., & Ganino, A. (1986). Interactive mismatch and repair: Challenges to the coping infant. *Zero to three, 6* (3), 1-6.

Tyack, D., & Gottsleben, R. (1975). *Language sampling analysis and training: A handbook for teachers and clinicians.* Palo Alto, CA: Consulting Psychology.

Uzgiris, I. C., & Hunt, J. (1975). *Assessment in infancy: Ordinal scales of psychological development.* Urbana: University of Illinois Press.

Watson, D. L., Omark, D. R., Grouell, S. T., & Heller, B. (1980). *Nondiscriminatory assessment: Practitioner's handbook,* Volume 1. Sacramento: California State Department of Education.

Weiss, H. B. (1988). Family support and education programs: The challenge and opportunities of an ecological approach. In H. Weiss & F. Jacobs (Eds.), *Evaluating family programs.* New York: Aldine.

Westby, C. (1980). Assessment of cognition and language abilities through play. *Journal of Language, Speech, and Hearing Services in the Schools, II,* 154–168.

Wolery, M., & Bailey, D., Jr. (1989). Assessing play skills. In D. Bailey, Jr., & M. Wolery (Eds.), *Assessing infants with handicaps* (pp. 428–446). New York: Merrill/Macmillan.

Yoder, D., & Kent, R. (1988). *Decision making in speech-language pathology.* Philadelphia, PA: B. C. Decker, Inc.

CHAPTER

5

MATCH-MISMATCH: A CLINICAL INTERVENTION MODEL

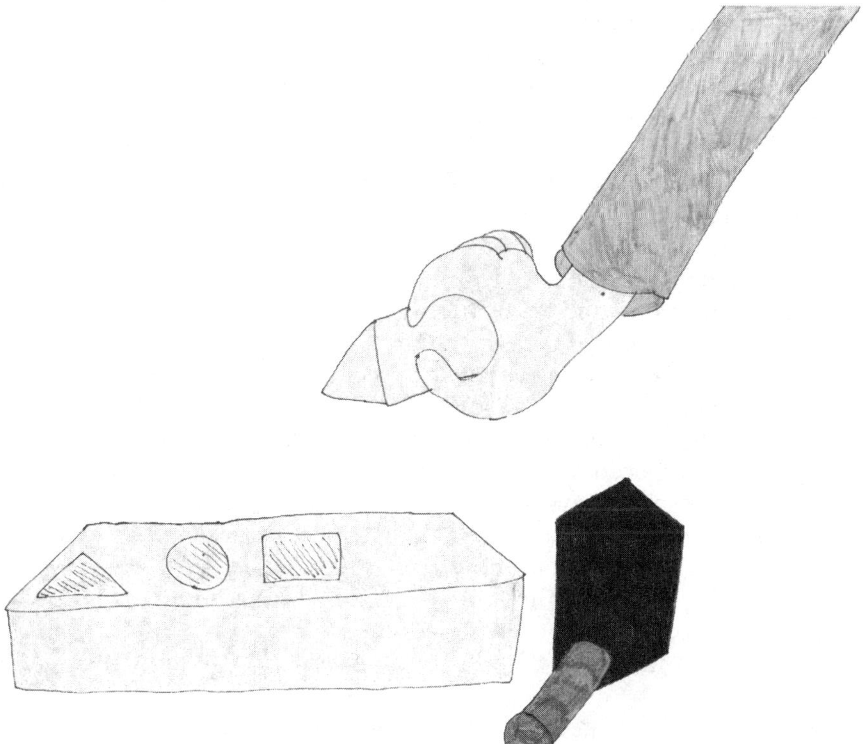

Matchmaker, Matchmaker
make me a match
find me a find
catch me a catch

Do you recognize these words from the musical *Fiddler on the Roof*? The singer is imploring the village matchmaker to find her a husband, someone who is just right for her. The matchmaker's job is quite an important one and she will work hard to find the right man for this woman. She must look closely at her to discover her strengths and weaknesses. She must perceive her as she is; then, with those perceptions she will work to find her a man who is well suited to her. Of course the matchmaker must know the qualities of the man as well. When the matchmaker has done her job well, the young woman and the young man will be a good match. They will meet each other's expectations; they will consider each other a good find, a good catch, a good fit.

What follows in this chapter is a saga of matchmaking. Our protagonists are teachers, parents, and children. What the authors hope to do is train you, the clinician, to be the matchmaker who facilitates the good match between the parent and the child, the parent and the teacher, the teacher and the child, and the child and the environment. It is not an easy task. Good therapeutic intervention is both a science and an art. Good matchmaking requires both science and art to find a good fit, to make a good match.

The purpose of this chapter is to present a clinical intervention model. The development of a clinical model is complex and difficult because there are always contributing variables that have been omitted. The purpose of a clinical model is to provide the clinician with a representational system that might highlight why therapeutic interaction does or does not operate effectively. Chess (1986) discussed a set of relationships that could contribute to an operational model in therapeutic intervention. The very idea that therapy can work when there is a synergy of variables provides a powerful tool for the young professional who needs to think about himself or herself, professional interactions, and clients and their families.

A clinical model allows the clinician to analyze ongoing therapeutic practice with the goal of evaluation and decision making in mind. It is only by means of self-analysis and self-investigation that the clinician has the ability to look back at what did not work and look forward with the goal of change. The clinical figure proposed by Chess (1986), representing "the goodness of fit concept," was utilized as a starting point in the framework of this chapter. In each section that follows, a figure representation will be generated, describing the match and mismatch possibilities. The purpose of the representations is to visually highlight for the student and the educator a feedback system in communication that can be utilized to analyze the interactional process between participants in therapy. When utilizing this model one must understand that

This chapter was co-authored by Dr. Christine Radziewicz.

the relationships are synergistic and constantly changing. When the synergy is cooperative and positively interactive, the total effect of the interaction is greater than the sum of the two effects taken independently.

In order to understand the process, it is important to understand the variables that affect the interactional dynamics. The perceptual variable in Figure 5-1 relates to the beliefs of an individual approaching a problem that needs to be resolved. These beliefs, which are often based on old information and past experiences, result in a cumulative framework that orients his or her viewpoint. The individual's expectations are generated by perceptions when he or she enters a novel situation. His or her beliefs create particular expectations in terms of (a) people's behaviors, (b) the outcome of events, and (c) the sequence of events.

When perceptions and expectations match the realities of an environmental occurrence, there is a synchrony or confluence that flows from perceptions to expectations to environmental occurrence. When there is a mismatch between perceptions/expectations and the reality of an environmental occurrence, there is a dissonance that requires resolution. The parties involved must each return to the source of the disharmony. Are one's beliefs incorrect? Are the expectations unrealistic? How do each of these influence the dissonance between the individual and the event? The clinical match requires some self-analysis, self-investigation, and self-inquiry. Sometimes the dissonance cannot be easily resolved because two people are diametrically opposed in their perceptions and are unwilling to alter their viewpoints of the situation. There are times when resolution cannot be accomplished, and it is our ability to accept the fact that we cannot agree that achieves the first step in conflict resolution. Perhaps time intervention and personal relationships create the catalyst for change in one or both individuals, and there is finally a shift in perceptual attitudes.

PARENT-CHILD INTERACTION

"Goodness of fit" is an early concept developed by Henderson in 1913. It relates to factors of consonance and dissonance between an organism and its environment. When the capacities, characteristics, and behaviors of an organism are in accord with the expectations of its environment, consonance occurs. When those capacities, characteristics, and behaviors are not in accord with the expectations of its environment, dissonance occurs. This model has been expanded by Chess and Thomas (1978) to account for outcomes of parent-child interactions. When the parents of a child have expectations and make demands that are in concert with the child's developmental potentials and capabilities, constructive interactions occur that result in growth and positive behaviors. When the parents' demands and expectations are beyond the capabilities of the child, distorted development and maladaptive functioning occurs. This "poorness of fit" situation implies that the demands, stresses, and conflicts that are inevitable and necessary for development in parent-child interactions are

Figure 5-1
Match = Consonance; Mismatch = Dissonance

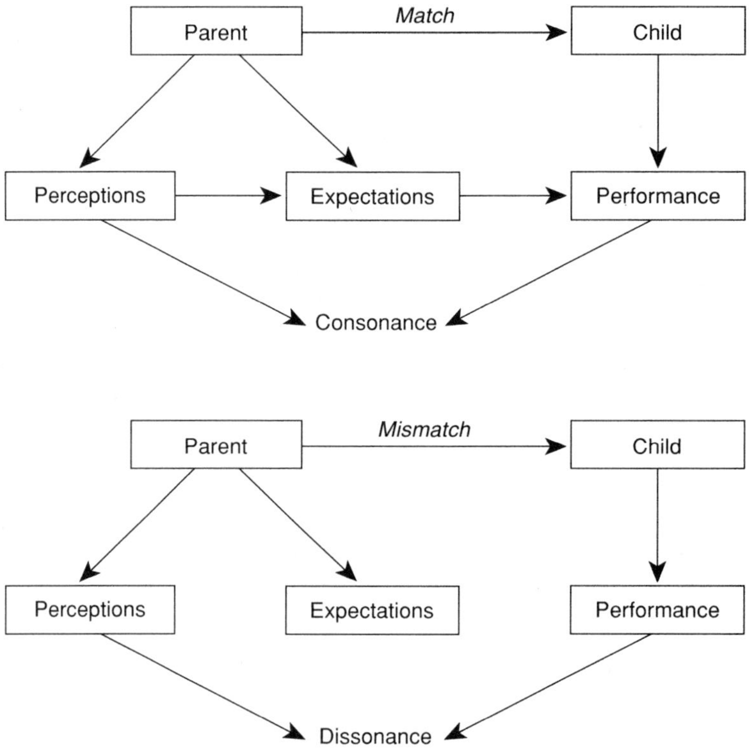

beyond the child's adaptive capacities. Just as Piaget proposed that cognitive growth is an outcome of a series of equilibrium and disequilibrium cycles, Chess and Thomas propose that patterns of behavior are an outcome of either good fit or poor fit between a child's characteristics and the parents' functioning. This section, Parent-Child Interaction, includes a number of variables. These variables lead to either consonance or dissonance. Figure 5-1 is a figural representation describing the match-mismatch possibilities that may occur between parent and child as they interact. Match results in an environment of consonance; mismatch results in an environment of dissonance. The variables that follow may be considered factors that affect the outcome of effective therapeutic intervention.

Linguistic Complexity

Linguistic complexity relates to a structural variable that may affect effective communication between parent and child. If linguistic complexity is appropriately regulated, the parent is able to match his or her level of information-input to the child's level of understanding. If the adult does not appropriately regulate the structure of information-input to the child's level of comprehension, the child does not understand, and a mismatch occurs. It is often the case that parents of language-disordered children do not effectively regulate the complexity of their input, which results in an obvious mismatch in communication between the parent and the child. When the adult's structures are complex and embedded, and the child's structures are emerging, there is little opportunity for the adult and the child to communicate effectively with each other. The matching process can only be accomplished when the parent and the child interact at similar linguistic levels. Parents must be taught to understand the child's linguistic structures and to tune in to the changing levels of linguistic learning. This would allow the adult to regulate down and up as a function of the child's level of performance. The language-disordered child does not have the ability to regulate his or her own language; therefore, adults and peers in the environment must make accommodations to the child's level of understanding. This means that parents must learn to listen to their language-disordered preschool child and match the adult structure to the child structure. This does not mean to imply that the adult is going to remain at the child's level. Here facilitation comes from the match and then the model. When the adult matches to the child's level of complexity, or linguistic structure, and then provides a more sophisticated production, the child has an opportunity to understand and progress. The more sophisticated model used by the parent is still reduced in terms of length and complexity and is often repeated and paraphrased, but it has been regulated to meet the capabilities of the child. When parents match their output to the capacities of the child it implies a sensitivity to and acceptance of the child's communicative style.

When a mismatch occurs between parent and child, the clinician working with them has an opportunity to step back from the clinical process and determine which variable must be manipulated to create a parent-child match. In order to accomplish this goal, the clinician must review the interactional process (see Figure 5-2). The variable that requires change might be linguistic complexity or the parent's interactive style. This figure suggests that the parents' perception of the child creates a set of expectations of the child's performance. When that performance does not meet the parents' expectations an opportunity arises for the parents to evaluate their perceptions and change their expectations. In terms of linguistic complexity, it was noted above that parents of children with language disorders often utilize complex linguistic structures without regard to the child's level of comprehension. Parents need to understand how much their children understand. One way to do this is to view the child realistically in a natural setting and compare his or her production abilities to his or her comprehension abilities. Parents often make incorrect assumptions about how much their children understand. In viewing the child in a natural setting, parents have an opportunity to view the child's language performance, change their perceptions of the child's language ability, and thus

Figure 5-2
Analyzing a Match: Adult-Child Interaction

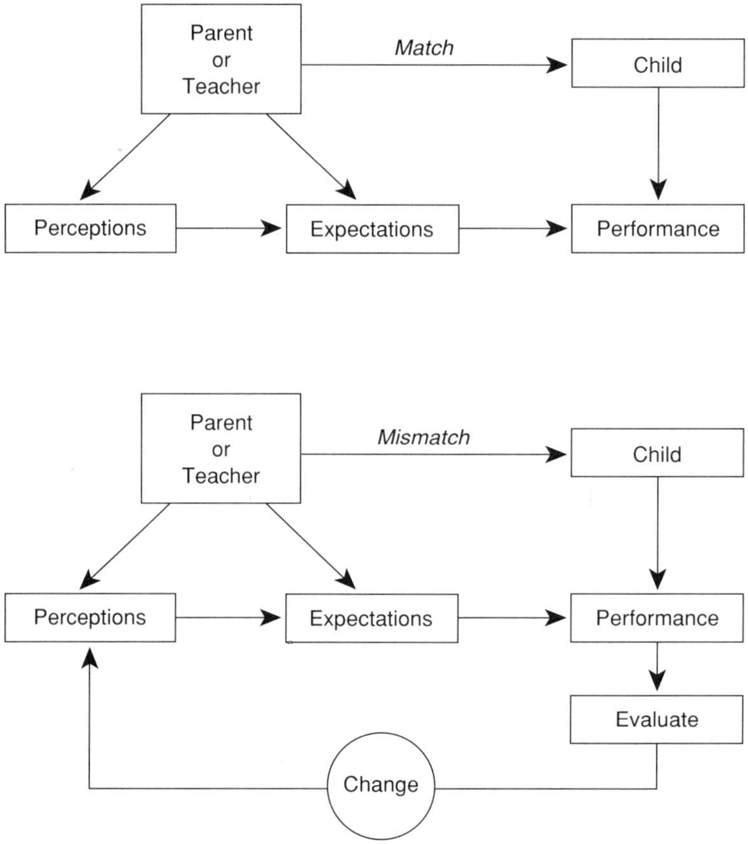

regulate the level of their linguistic complexity down to the child's level of understanding. Tiegerman and Siperstein (1984) describe the fact that parents of language-disordered children with an MLU of 1.0 often utilize complex structures of 15.0 morphemes or more. Clearly, there is a mismatch between the adult structures and the child's ability to understand those structures. These researchers also describe the fact that parents of language-disordered children utilize monologue role structures with a high frequency of questions. The impact communicatively is that the adult asks the child a question and then answers it without allowing the child the opportunity to provide either a nonverbal or a verbal response. In questioning parents about the use of questions, this population of mothers indicated that over time they realized that they could not have a conversation with their children, so they asked questions and did not expect responses. The mismatch here is obviously the fact that the expectation is that the child is not going to respond or cannot respond. The parent does not allow the child to respond or look to see if the child has responded. Mothers had to be trained to change their expectations and their interactional behaviors with their preschool children who had language disorders.

In terms of parental style, the mismatch might take the form of a parent's expectation that the child will approach new learning situations enthusiastically and boldly, similarly to the way the parent approaches them. However, if the child's pattern of behavior is one of caution and slow, measured exploration, there will be a mismatch of parent expectation and child performance. The parent may introduce a constant flow of new objects/materials/toys during play interactions, expecting them to enhance language learning. This parent may go on and on talking about and manipulating the toys with the expectation that it will maximize the communicative process. The child who adapts slowly to novel items or situations is not able to easily integrate the verbal input and new physical environment easily. This child will probably not enjoy and luxuriate in this communicative interaction. The mismatch has resulted in a less than optimal opportunity for language learning. In this instance the clinician must enable the parent to accept and understand the mismatch of interactive style between her and the child. Neither the parent nor the child needs to be "fixed." What is needed is an adaptation of parental expectations and output to child's capacities and performance.

Semantic Relatedness

Snow and Ferguson (1977) proposed a semantic theory described earlier in the text as motherese that had important implications in child language. The basic tenet of semantic relatedness is the matching process itself. In being semantically related to the child, the parent regulates the content of his or her productions, not the form. The child sets the topic and the parent provides information on that topic so long as the child remains interested. Parents of normal language learners are semantically related approximately 70 percent of the time. During conversational exchange, this provides a high degree of communicative and semantic matching that is language-rich in its instructional content. The adult talks about what the child is doing and/or saying as the child is engaged in environmental experiences. This means that the child has a running commentary about the environment. The language immersion experience is child-centered, child-oriented, and child-focused. The adult's intent is clearly to provide the child with as much information and knowledge about the world as possible. A match exists when the parents' linguistic output is appropriate to the capacities of the child.

If the child is playing with trucks and Mother is providing information about dolls, the child is not likely to integrate much of what Mother is saying because his or her interests are elsewhere. Mother must learn to watch and engage the child when he or she is interested and motivated. Figure 5-2 shows the potential mismatch between parent and child. If the mother is not focused on the child's interactional performance in a context, her language behaviors may not reflect the child's interests or actions. The mismatch here is the mother's perceptions and expectations of what the child's communicative interactive performance should be. The result is a missed or lost opportunity for semantic learning; the child is playing with one object and the parent is talking about another. Clearly, if the child does not respond to the mother's verbal or nonverbal behavior, Mother must then evaluate her expectations of the child, critically looking at the child, his or her play behavior, and the objects that he or she is manipulating and comparing the contextual occurrence to her linguistic output. If her input is not matched to the context, her perceptions and expectations of the child's abilities do not match his or her performance. A closer look at the child's performance results in an evaluation of the mother's language behavior that would lead to a change in her perceptions of what the child's needs are. This then would result in a change in her language input and a change in her perceptions and expectations of the child's performance. Thus a match is facilitated.

Family Attitudes

Most parents do not have prior knowledge when it comes to identifying a language-disordered child. Parents are often shocked, disillusioned, and frightened. Their belief that they have a perfect child is shattered; now they must come to terms with reality. Parents have many misconceptions about disabled children. One advantage to early identification through Public Law 99-457 is that family issues and concerns are addressed as early as possible in the developmental process. Professionals must dispel the family's misconceptions and misperceptions. Children develop best when their values and assets are recognized. Family members who do not perceive the children realistically become frustrated; their anxiety changes to the misperception that such children cannot learn. The earlier the problem is identified, the greater will be the opportunity for the family to come to terms with their attitudes about having a disabled child. There may be cultural variations that overprotect the child or reject him or her completely. Neither of these are productive in today's society. The educational philosophy in the United States rejects the idea that children be warehoused or institutionalized because they are disabled; disabled children cannot be segregated from society. Clearly, the first line of integration must come from within the family. The emotional match that will result in growth and fulfillment of potential is one of acceptance—the acceptance of the child in the family. The stronger the rejection, the greater the conflict between the child and the family and among family members. The mismatch within the family relates to the parents' negative perceptions of the disabled child—their disappointment and disillusionment. The family has difficulty understanding that a disabled child can and will learn, and can become competent if he or she is helped to realize his or her potential.

Figure 5-2 shows that children must be viewed realistically; they must be "measured" in terms of their own abilities and not compared to older or younger siblings. Mismatches can be changed to matches only when parents and other family members do not see children in terms of their disabilities. When they are helped to evaluate the child realistically, they come to understand that he or she has the potential to learn. As the child learns, the family develops more realistic expectations of what and how he or she can accomplish at home and in school. This match between parent and child allows for the family to integrate the child so that he or she can function as a participating member of the family. Another form of mismatch can occur between family and child when the family overestimates the capabilities of the child. The child experiences stress because his or her performance never matches the expectations of the family; both family and child feel frustration. Often the parents' misperceptions of the child's abilities and performance prevent them from seeking the professional help and services that are sorely needed by the child.

Family Economy

Families of disabled children are often faced with exorbitant medical bills and expenses. The stress of having children with no special needs is difficult enough in today's society. The introduction of a disabled child into the family adds additional economic stress. The mismatch between parent and child includes the shock of the financial stress and the negative feelings related to the additional burden. Often resources must be shifted from the other children to the disabled child. There are natural resentments that must be addressed as parents turn away from each other and from the other children to take care of the needs of the disabled child. A match can occur only if parents see the immediate stress as a short-term crisis and recognize that there are support systems that must be developed outside of the immediate family. Relatives, respite programs, educational programs, family counseling, and private therapy are all mechanisms to support the family and enable all of the members to deal with the economic crisis. Parents must learn to evaluate their resources in terms of this short-term crisis and change their negative perceptions to more realistic long-term goals. They must learn to change their roles and expectations of each other. Clearly, the expectation that only the father functions as the breadwinner is not realistic. The father must change his expectation of his role and his wife's role in the family. The mother must learn to see herself as an active working contributor and allow her husband to function in more direct childcare responsibilities. Clearly, the demands of the "financial crunch" in the family will demand a change in gender roles, gender rules, and gender responsibilities. The match will occur only if parents are able to alter their perceptions and expectations of each other so that they are able to mobilize their resources to meet the needs of the disabled child and the financial stability in the family.

Family Health

The ability of the family to survive the crisis of a disabled child begins with the initial steps of acknowledgment and acceptance—acceptance that the preschool child is in fact a special learner. David Luterman (1979) reports that the initial experience of parents of a disabled child is predictable and universal; their psychological reaction to the realization that their child is disabled is one of grief and mourning, similar to the reaction described by Elizabeth Kubler-Ross (1969). This reaction is grouped into stages: shock, recognition, denial, acknowledgment, and creative action. Shock and recognition are short-term stages, but denial can be long-term, can take many forms, and frequently manifests itself as anger. The stage of acknowledgment brings with it acceptance of the child and the handicap; frequently parents in this stage are ready to meet with other parents of disabled children and talk freely and openly about their child's special needs. Constructive action is the final stage of the mourning process; at this time the parents are ready to re-examine their value systems and expectations. It is in this stage that parents are ready to enhance the learning experiences of their child. The health of the family involves its emotional well-being and its ability to survive and manage the long-term effects of having a disabled child. The family needs to evaluate its emotional strengths and weaknesses; its members need to discuss how each person feels about the child and about other family members. The mismatch in the family relates to the negative perceptions and disappointments related to having a disabled child. Parents might be angry and frustrated; they might feel guilty or that they are being punished by God. They talk about their disillusionment: "I thought I was having a perfect child." "Will I ever have grandchildren?"

Having a disabled child means coming to terms with the life cycle process. Parents must evaluate their perceptions and expectations and ultimately change through acceptance. When they learn to accept the child for who he or she is, there is no conflict and no anger. They must learn to help each other and help the other siblings so that there is no guilt or shame. Support groups and family counseling are particularly helpful in teaching members of the family to talk to each other and communicate their feelings about the disabled child and each other. Members of the family must learn to support each other emotionally so that each member makes a contribution.

Family Structure and Roles

The traditional American family—two parents and two children—is no longer representative of today's families. Within the structure of that traditional family, the father had a primary dominant role and responsibility as the breadwinner. The mother had a primary responsibility in the home, did not work outside the home, and took care of all of the child-care responsibilities and duties. One of the issues that is often raised about the traditional family in American society and sociologically across cultures is that when roles and structures are clearly defined, there are fewer conflicts between adults. It is also apparently the case that when the roles are clearly defined in the home and outside of the home, there are fewer gender-based problems in terms of "what fathers do" and "what mothers do."

The economic pressures in today's society have resulted in a blurring of family structure, roles, and responsibilities. Perhaps the most significant changes relate to the fact that in the twenty-first century, the American workforce will be heavily represented by women, many of them mothers. In fact, by the year 2000, 87 percent of all mothers will have work-related responsibilities outside the home. If mothers are working outside the home, to what extent does the home context change to reflect the demands of their working responsibilities and/or professional requirements? Do perceptions and expectations remain the same for both parents or is there a need for reevaluation and change of these perceptions and expectations?

In Chapter 6, Training the Parent as Facilitator, Figure 6-2, mothers and fathers were polled to determine their attitudes and concerns about child-care issues as they affected the disabled child. Fathers expressed the attitude that child raising was primarily the mother's responsibility; mothers indicated that coping with the stresses of working outside the home did not give them the time, the inclination, or the emotional wherewithal to manage all of the duties related to child care. Clearly, the addition of a youngster with a disability to the family adds a burden to traditional family structures and roles and presents serious problems that cannot be addressed with traditional attitudes, perceptions, and expectations.

The mismatch in the family relates to the fact that if parents have expectations of each other that do not result in a supportive function for the child, there will be conflict between the adults as to who is responsible for taking care of the child. The disabled child is not just one person's responsibility; he or she is everyone's responsibility. Each member of the family has a role to play in supporting and nurturing the child's growth and development. The question is, does the family have the internal resources to assess their own strengths and weaknesses and effect changes in order to accomplish this goal?

The purpose of a family assessment is in fact to determine the strength of each family member and to identify each person's contribution. Family members must understand that the family structure and roles might need to be changed so that each person receives some relief and respite and no one, particularly the mother, is the sole caretaker or carries the primary burden. By means of a family assessment, a match can be achieved; realistic perceptions will result in realistic expectations of each family member in relation to each other and to the disabled child. The difference in perception must be bridged in order to facilitate family change and family cohesion.

Behavioral Considerations

Ongoing behavioral difficulties present one of the most pressing problems for parents of preschool children with disabilities. Parents are often mortified by temper tantrums and inappropriate behaviors that are exhibited in public places. It becomes very difficult to take the child to a restaurant, a grocery store, or a shopping center because he or she is "unmanageable and uncooperative." Here the mismatch relates to the fact that parents perceive the child's behavior as willful and manipulative and expect that he or she should behave or should know better.

Parents need to understand that children's behavioral performances relate specifically to their ability or inability to understand the social context. As children's language becomes more sophisticated and complex, they become more capable of socialization and of acting more appropriately in social contexts. Parents also need to understand that in evaluating children's performance, they need to evaluate the challenge of the context.

It may not be appropriate to take a child to a large shopping center after school when he or she is tired. Parents must assess what the child's capabilities are and then evaluate the context in relation to the social demands. This might mean changing schedules and making arrangements based on the child's abilities. During the course of the day, parents must learn to be flexible and supportive of each other. The shopping trip might be put off for another time, or one parent or the other might volunteer to shop without the child. The match occurs when parents realistically assess the child's performance during the course of the day and then make adjustments between child demands and family routines.

Summary: Match-Mismatch

The attitudes and perceptions of the family play a critical role in the child's progress in school. The family must learn to assess realistically not only the child's needs, but also his or her ability to progress and change. Parents and other family members can acquire the necessary understanding and knowledge of the child's language-learning difficulties by attending parent training class, reading therapeutic materials, and seeking counseling services. All of these activities will help to establish realistic goals for the child in his or her natural environment—the home.

Accepting the child for "who his is" and "where he is" allows the family and all of its members to move forward in their own growth and development. The denial of the child's needs serves only to hinder his or her progress and sometimes interferes with the intervention process itself. In accepting the child, the family accepts the reality of the problem and seeks ways to mobilize in support of the child's growth and development. In accepting the child, the focus is on change rather than denial. The family must come to terms with a match between the child's language-learning needs, their perceptions of the child, and the reality of special education.

TEACHER-PARENT INTERACTION

This section deals with the fact that in attempting to change child behaviors, parents and teachers must learn to communicate with each other about their perceptions and expectations. The variables in this section reflect some factors that may influence differences between parents and teachers that affect their

Figure 5-3
Analyzing a Match: Adult-Adult Interaction

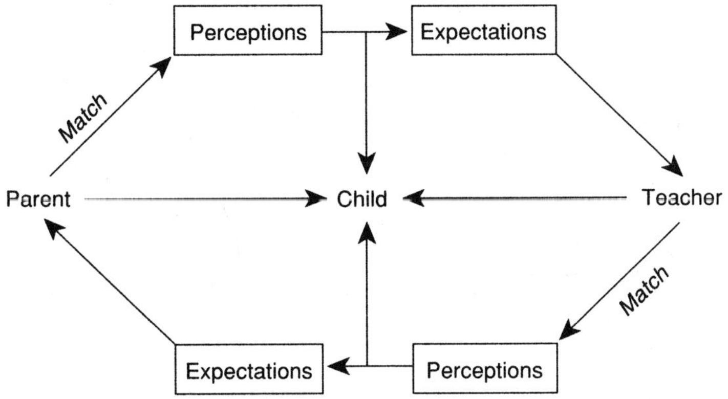

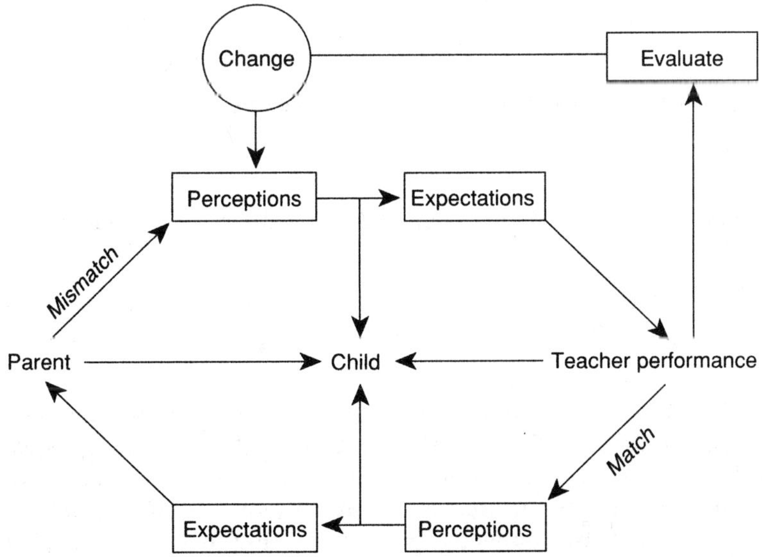

Example of 1 Mismatch

Figure 5-4
Analyzing a Triadic Interaction

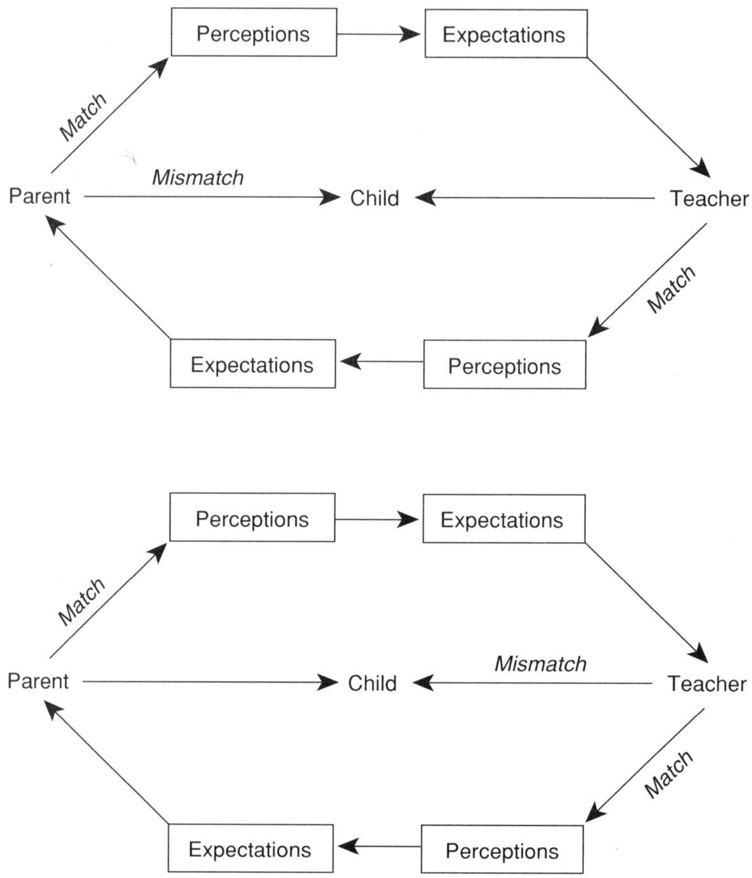

ability to understand each other and to understand the child (see Figures 5-3 and 5-4).

Education

The difference in educational training and abilities between parents and teachers represents a significant problem. A mismatch will occur in communication if teachers expect parents of preschool children to have a complete understanding of their child and possible concomitant learning problems; a mismatch will also occur if parents expect teachers to know everything. Another problem arises if the parent perceives the child to be at one developmental level and the teacher perceives the child to be at another. The reality is that the parent must evaluate the teacher's context and understanding of the child based on classroom experiences; the teacher must evaluate the parent's knowledge of the child based on home experiences. It is also important for teachers to keep in mind that parents do not have formalized educational training in the field of developmental disabilities and to take the time to increase the parents' knowledge base by inviting them into the classroom, by offering educational training classes, and by providing the necessary emotional support. Figure 5-3 describes the match-mismatch possibility in the interactional exchange between parents and teachers. Differences in education present an immediate problem. Teachers are formally educated about developmental disabilities; parents are not. When parents and teachers, therefore, come together, they might recognize their educational differences, but they must give each other credit for different experiences, different perceptions, and different interactions with the child.

Multicultural Issues

Multicultural influences are dramatically changing American society. Cities across the United States are faced with the difficult demands of educating culturally different children from all over the world. Cultural diversity issues include language or dialect differences, family differences, and childrearing differences. Differences in language and in cultural perspectives create significant problems in parent-teacher communication and greatly influence how parents and teachers interact. Teachers who are trained in the American educational system might feel that that system provides the best learning mechanism for all children. Parents from different cultures have different perspectives and values and obviously require different educational curricula than those that presently exist. The multicultural school cannot present a single approach to educating disabled and nondisabled children.

Minority parents feel that their cultural values should be reflected in the educational system and process in their community school. The clash between American-educated teachers and minority parents is a real threat to the accomplishment of educational programming for all children. A mismatch occurs when parents from multicultural backgrounds perceive that teachers do not understand their values and have expectations that teachers need to teach differently. Another mismatch occurs when teachers perceive that parents from minority backgrounds do not have the skills or abilities to educate or make educational decisions about their children and therefore expect that parents will play a passive role in the educational process. A match can only occur if parents and teachers learn to understand what the multicultural issues are and how these differences can provide a bridge to facilitate change. Miller (1984) suggests that some of the multicultural related factors that are at risk for creating a mismatch include childrearing practices, reaction to confrontation, sociocultural position, societal role, test-taking attitudes, adjustment to artificiality of tests, use of culture-bound stimuli, conceptual differences, selection practices for determining normative samples, and judgment questions. When parents and teachers are aware of these differences they can change their perceptions and expectations of each other. They can accept the validity of different values and beliefs and integrate them into the parent-teacher relationship. The reality is that multicultural differences can enrich educational curricula for all children—disabled and nondisabled.

Religious Affiliation

The role of religion in the public schools remains a highly controversial issue in today's society. The diversity of religious groups also presents potential problems in educational development and in parent-teacher interaction. This can best be highlighted by the fact that many public school districts have developed seasonal activities that reflect multicultural and religious references. Some religious groups and nonreligious groups such as atheists object to the use of seasonal and/or religious terms and foods in educational activities. These biases obviously create a mismatch between parent and teacher in the development of educational curricula in the course of the year. Some parents have perceptions and expectations that their religious belief or any religious belief cannot be discussed or represented in a public school. Other parents feel very strongly about the development and infusion of religious issues in the public domain. A match can only occur with the development of tolerance on all sides, given the demands of educational programming for children with disabilities. Very often parents and teachers lose site of the first priority—to educate the disabled preschool child.

Parental Involvement

Chapter 6 deals extensively with parent education. The role of the parent is not clearly defined in either Public Law 94-142 or Public Law 99-457. The term *parental involvement* is used in the laws and in state regulations; however, what *parental involvement* means specifically depends on the school district, the professionals involved, and the willingness of the parents to advocate for their child.

A mismatch occurs when a teacher feels that a parent is too pushy or doesn't listen or is too involved—or feels that a parent is not involved, doesn't care, and does not show up in school. A mismatch can also occur when a parent feels locked out of the educational system because there are no formal classes, no mechanism to observe the child in the classroom, and no understanding of family cultural or educational values. In all these instances the mismatch is due to incongruence of perceptions and expectations with performance. Obviously change must occur. This change requires an adjustment in perceptions and expectations on the part of teachers and parents.

A match can only occur if parents and teachers meet formally to develop a set of parent-teacher rights that clearly defines the roles of the parent and the teacher and the ways they must collaborate to accommodate educational goals. This would also facilitate development of parent education programs that would enable families to contribute more effectively and efficiently to the educational development of their children at home.

Attitudes: Negative and Positive

In Chapter 7, The Classroom as Language Laboratory, the issue of attitude is described in terms of parent and teacher expectations and parent and teacher differences. Without a doubt, parents and teachers begin the school year with a whole set of attitudes that relate specifically to past experiences. If they have had positive experiences with each other in the past, their attitudes will be positive toward each other in the future. If they have had negative experiences with each other in the past, those negative attitudes will also be rolled forward. Teachers who perceive parents as lazy, limited, or hostile will have negative expectations of parental behavior and negative expectations in terms of the child.

It is often difficult for teachers to separate the parent from the child. Parents who have had negative experiences with teachers automatically assume that the teacher will "take out" the problems on the child. These attitudes must be openly discussed because the child is the final product of the parent-teacher relationship. A match can occur only when parents and teachers discuss their perceptions of each other and their expectations in terms of the child. Parents and teachers must learn to view each other realistically to develop realistic expectations of the child's performances in the classroom and in the home.

Summary: Match-Mismatch

American society is complicated by its changing multicultural influences. Our differences in perceptions and different beliefs present challenges to education and conflict resolution. The clinical match between teacher and parent can only be accomplished when we accept our differences and learn to negotiate a resolution. It is important for parents and teachers to acknowledge that each is doing a job and that they are each doing the best they possibly can.

Parents cannot be expected to be teachers, and teachers cannot be expected to be parents. The roles and responsibilities are interdependent, but they are not the same. Parents must learn to evaluate the teacher's performance, given the context of the classroom, which is a complex learning environment with many other children who have needs and demands. Parents must see and observe for themselves the complexities of the learning environment and the problems that the teacher faces in meeting the challenges of the classroom.

On the other hand, teachers must learn that parents are faced with a complicated and complex set of variables in the home environment. The pressures there are just as taxing and exhausting as the challenges of the classroom. Although the needs and dynamics may be different in each of these environments, a healthy respect for each other's role goes a long way in achieving a mutual understanding of the differences that face all of us.

TEACHER-CHILD INTERACTION

This section discusses the dynamic interaction that occurs in the classroom between teacher and child. Figure 5-2 can be used to describe the interactional variables that occur in the match-mismatch process. In the framework of the classroom group experience, the teacher must meet the language and social needs of the group *and* the individual language and social needs of each child in the group. The challenge is to identify a mean group language level and facilitate language learning in the group so that each child achieves that level.

Linguistic Regulation

The teacher, like the parent, must regulate the form and the content of his or her input to the child's level of comprehension and provide a language-learning model that is semantically related to the child's experiential knowledge, thereby facilitating a scaffolding framework. In the group, children function at different language levels. In addition, they do not present with the same language-learning abilities across the component areas of pragmatics, semantics, syntax, and phonology. This means that just as the children in the group may have different linguistic abilities, they also have different language profiles. The task for the teacher is to individualize his or her input to each child, with that child's linguistic level and language profile in mind. One technique that can be used to accomplish this goal is for the teacher to facilitate the interaction between two children, to engage them in a dyadic verbal and/or nonverbal interaction. The teacher monitors the interchange, filling in the interactional spaces by modeling appropriate language behaviors. The primary goal is to reinforce each child's interactional behavior and extend the number of communicative turns on a topic.

Figure 5-2 highlights the fact that the teacher must be aware of the group's linguistic level as well as each child's level in order to create a communicative match. A mismatch occurs when the teacher cannot facilitate an interaction between two children because their communicative abilities cannot be bridged by the activity or by modeling. Each child's ability must be accurately assessed for there to be a good communicative fit between children. Working with communication partners and buddies allows children to develop successful language and interactional exchanges. This practice with partners enables them to acquire specific skills. Once these specific conversational skills are acquired in the interactional repertoire, these behaviors can be generalized to other communicative partners. The initial matching in a classroom occurs then between children. The teacher can develop a list of communicative partner dyads based on the type of classroom activity, allowing children to practice specific skills with different language partners. Understanding each child's language needs becomes the pivotal factor in establishing the dyadic match. Figure 5-5 can be used to chart the communicative functioning level of each child in the classroom. It will provide a "communication map" that will enable the teacher to match communication behaviors of children in the classroom and to recognize when bridging by modeling is necessary. The specific language behaviors listed in Figure 5-5 are just some of the behaviors that can be documented; it is not a complete listing. However, the purpose of this communication map is to list those target behaviors that children in one classroom have in common.

When a communication breakdown occurs between children, the teacher must analyze the interactional exchange to determine the nature of the breakdown. Since the children are language disordered, they will not be able to engage in any metalinguistic repair work. The teacher will have to revise and repair the communicative exchange to reestablish the verbal and/or nonverbal conversational interaction. Facilitating each child to function appropriately in the roles of speaker and listener provides for experiential learning. Children learn by doing; they can only learn to have a conversation by actually engaging in the process. This is particularly difficult for the language-disordered child who does not have the skills to initiate or to maintain the interactional process and therefore does not learn by himself or herself. The language-disordered preschooler must be provided with the scaffolding—the opportunity, the framework, and the instructional guidance to interact and to learn about the conversational process.

Teacher Facilitation Techniques

In attempting to facilitate child-language development as well as child socialization, the classroom teacher utilizes a number of different techniques. One such technique, described above, is for the teacher to act as director or facilitator between two children who have been matched in terms of their language-learning abilities. The teacher reinforces individual interactional skills in each child and maintains a social communicative exchange between the two children. In attempting to accomplish this goal, the teacher can use an imitation technique that would require, in the course of a communicative breakdown, one child to imitate the teacher's language model. Another technique is the use of a partial model in which the teacher provides part of a sentence, word, or structure that would be imitated to continue and/or reestablish the communicative exchange between children. A third technique would be for the teacher to ask one of the children a specific question, the response to which would facilitate

Figure 5-5
Mapping the Communication Needs of Children within a Classroom

Children	Pragmatic				Semantic				Other	
	Turntaking	Appropriate eye gaze	Physical proxemics	Requests	Regulates	Protests	Calls attention	Answers/ responds	MLU Range	
1. John D.	DL	DL	A	ND	ND	DL				
2. Mary B.	DL	DL	DL	DL	DL	DA				
3. Jose G.	DL	ND	DL	ND	ND	DL				
4. Carol N.	DA	DA	DA	ND	DL	DA				
5.										
6.										
7.										
8.										
9.										
10.										
11.										
12.										

DA - Demonstrated/Adequate DL - Demonstrated/Limited
ND - Not Demonstrated A - Appropriate

interaction, verbal or nonverbal, between the two children. Expansion is a fourth technique that readily lends itself to facilitating child-child interaction. The teacher expands on a child's communication to another child in order to match the first child's communicative attempt with the understanding level of the second child.

These facilitation techniques can be expanded to include the dyadic exchange, a triadic exchange, and progressively a larger group interaction in the remaining work of a larger group experience. One important dynamic is to teach each child to function as a speaker and as a listener in the group. As a result, each child must learn not only to take his or her turn but also to wait for his or her turn to communicate. Activities such as show and tell and calendar can be utilized to teach specific roles and rules of language interaction in a group setting.

The teacher must establish a mean language level for the group. Some of the children will be able to express sophisticated language productions; the productions of others will be more limited. The result, however, will be that each child has an opportunity to function in the group and contribute to the group language activity. The matching process in this situation must be progressive in nature. This means that the dynamics occurring in a small dyadic exchange will be much more enhanced, magnified, and complex in a large group activity; the skills must be developed first in the dyad and then generalized to the larger group experience. The matching process occurs when the classroom teacher identifies the appropriate mean language level for the group and then facilitates the development of each child's language so that his or her performance approximates that mean language level. Utilizing the communication map (see Figure 5-5) will enable the teacher to establish a mean language level and match each child's level with the group mean level. A mismatch will occur if the child is placed in a large group experience and then cannot meet the challenge of roles and rules in the group. The teacher must provide an interim experience by limiting the group size and then working specifically on the skills that the child needs to function as a speaker and as a listener in a large group.

Behavioral Considerations

Very often preschool children with severe language and communication disorders present with a range of behavior symptomatology, from withdrawal to aggressive hitting or biting. These behaviors, which often appear in a group situation during individual instruction or when the teacher-child level of interaction is highly structured and frequent, can be minimized by means of various reinforcement techniques and cues provided to the child. It is important for the teacher to understand, to note, and to collect data on the activities that present the most difficulty for children with behavioral symptomatology. If the teacher sits next to or behind the language-disordered child, he or she has an opportunity to manage disruptive behaviors that occur when the child does not understand and therefore becomes distracted and frustrated. A more appropriate setting for a child with behavioral needs is in a small group context, which allows a high degree of structure and a high degree of adult input. Often children cannot manage each other; when Michael hits Susie, Susie becomes reluctant to interact with Michael in the future. This is a clear example of a social mismatch that must be rectified by facilitating more appropriate social communicative and behavioral interaction between the two children. Interestingly, children with behavioral needs desperately need the experiences of the group setting. With severe behavioral symptomatology, however, they rule themselves out of the very settings that they need. The match can be accomplished when the teacher becomes aware of Michael's preliminary behavioral agitations and redirects him to a smaller group setting and/or another activity before he exhibits aggressive behavior. A match can also be accomplished when a more sophisticated language peer can be utilized to engage Michael in appropriate verbal and/or nonverbal activities. Both children can then be reinforced for appropriate interactions: Michael for exhibiting appropriate social behaviors and remaining engaged in an exchange, and the peer for facilitating Michael's behavior. Again, the technique of modeling can be utilized to encourage a peer to initiate and maintain interaction with Michael.

Teaching Style vs. Learning Style

It has often been noted in the literature that classroom teachers, as a function of their personality, their training, and their observations of children, utilize highly individualized instructional styles. In teaching, it has also been noted that preschool language-disordered children, like many other language learners, have preferences in learning about their environment and the world around them. A mismatch can occur when the teacher's style of facilitation conflicts with the child's style of learning. Teachers must learn how the child acquires knowledge in the classroom. If the child is more visually based, or auditorily based, or kinesthetically based, accommodations must be made in the way in which activities are presented and input is provided. Likewise the teacher must take into account other attributes and styles of each child—activity level, distractibility, persistence, attention span, willingness to approach novel tasks and situations, and adaptability. The teacher must match activities and their duration and physical setting to the style of the child.

The classroom teacher can learn about the child's learning style simply by observing him or her with objects, during free play, and during interaction with peers. A child's social and communicative style will become quite evident; stylistic issues can become educational considerations. The teacher can organize and document a child's learning style by charting the behaviors observed in different contexts as shown in Figure 5-6, then using the resulting map to generate activities that match the child's learning style. For instance, if a child is somewhat distractible, has a moderate activity level, and responds best to visual and kinesthetic/tactile cues, a learning activity that incorporates move-

Figure 5-6
Learning Style Map

	Always	Often	Sometimes	Never
Distractible				
High activity level				
Moderate activity level				
Low activity level				
Persistent				
Attentive				
Approaches novel situations readily				
Responds to auditory cueing to facilitate learning				
Responds to visual cueing to facilitate learning				
Responds to tactile/kinesthetic cues to facilitate learning				
Adapts to routine changes				

ment and various textured materials would be best. Any activity that requires long waiting time between turns and doesn't include visual or tactile cues would be inappropriate and definitely mismatched to this child's style.

Teacher Expectations and Perceptions

At the beginning of the school year, all classroom teachers have expectations of their own performance and their children's accomplishments. Preschool children with language disorders very often make small but steady changes and steps in their growth and development. A mismatch can occur when a classroom teacher expects the preschool language-disordered child to grow and develop in a way in which a non–special-needs child might. The teacher must carefully observe the children in the classroom and view their accomplishments and changes in order to establish appropriate goals; a teacher who comes into the classroom with preestablished activities and goals is often met with frustration and failure. The process begins by observing the children and noting their language abilities. Based on individual abilities and the convergence of group abilities, the teacher can establish realistic activities and goals for the year. This establishes a more appropriate match between the teacher's expectations and the children's ultimate performances.

Summary: Match-Mismatch

The way in which children are labeled often does not qualitatively or quantitatively match the realities of their performance in school. Because labels leave a great deal to be desired in terms of elucidating skills, abilities, and achievements, teachers must learn to evaluate based on variables other than I.Q. and reading scores. The communicative and social variables that are developed in a classroom cannot be underestimated in terms of their application to real-world abilities. Teachers must learn to separate personal expectations from the realities of classroom dynamics. Although they might expect a particular skill to be acquired in a certain period of time, children will not acquire that skill in anything other than their own time framework.

Teachers must learn that a child is a teacher, and a child teaches. They must learn to take their cues, their clues, and their insights from their students. The classroom and the educational process need to be child-initiated and child-directed. It is not necessary to control every aspect of the classroom environment. An important clinical match occurs when teachers acknowledge that their central power comes from learning from students and that the student is the ultimate teacher.

A Few Words From Toya Davis

The idea of match-mismatch is an interesting one. We choose our friends and our mates based on those characteristics that seem to mesh best with our own. However, we certainly can't choose our children in the same way, and we certainly don't choose to have a disabled child. That's not to say that we don't love our disabled child with all our hearts. But it is true that we are not prepared for what lies ahead. We want what's best for the child, but we sometimes get burdened with frustration when he or she doesn't progress as we hoped, or meet our expectations. Fear can take its grip too. We fear that this child will never learn or function in society as we had expected. This can lead to an anger that can immobilize us. It is at these times that we need most to stop, reflect, analyze, and evaluate. It takes courage to do this. It takes courage to look at ourselves, to perceive ourselves as we really are, and to honestly look at our child and accept him for who he is. Maybe what we're doing is an attitude adjustment, or a perception and expectation adjustment. I've never gone to a chiropractor, but I believe that they provide a service called "adjustment." This "adjustment" aligns the spinal vertebrae so that the body can move comfortably and with ease. Perhaps that is what the perception/expectation adjustment will do for parents—enable them to align or match with the needs and strengths of their child and move through life with ease.

REFERENCES

Chess, S. (1986). Early childhood development and its implications for analytic theory and practice. *American Journal of Psychoanalysis, 46,* 122–148.

Chess, S., & Thomas, A. (1978). Temperamental traits and parent guidance. In E. Arnold (Ed.), *Helping parents help their children.* New York: Bruner/Mazel.

Henderson, L. V. (1913). *The fitness of the environment.* New York: Macmillan.

Kubler-Ross, E. (1969). *On death and dying.* New York: Macmillan.

Luterman, D. (1979). *Counseling parents of hearing impaired children.* Boston: Little Brown and Company.

Miller, L. (1984). Classroom based language intervention. *Language Speech Hearing Services in the Schools, 20,* 153–169.

Snow, C. E., & Ferguson, C. A. (Eds.) (1977). *Talking to children: Language input and acquisition.* Cambridge: Cambridge University Press.

Tiegerman, E., & Siperstein, M. (1984, September). Individual patterns of interaction in the mother-child dyad: Implications for parent intervention. *Topics in Language Disorders.*

CHAPTER

6

TRAINING THE PARENT AS FACILITATOR

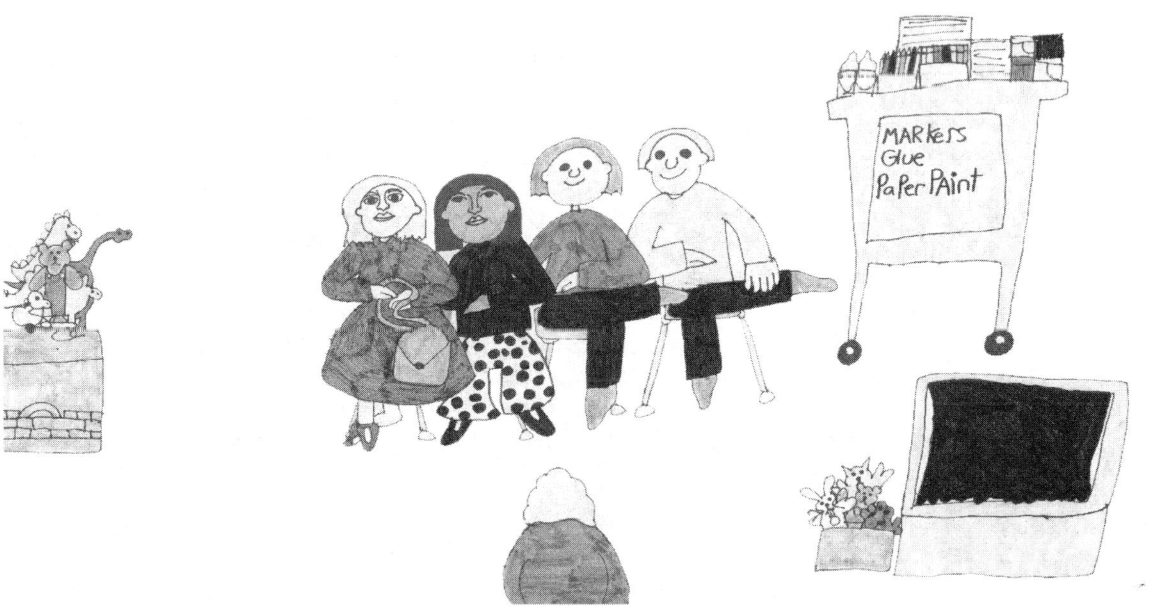

One of the primary issues discussed in Chapter 2, The Changing Role of the Family, involved the role of the parents in the education of the children with disabilities. Clearly, parents have felt disenfranchised from the educational process. Given the needs of preschool children with language disorders, interestingly enough, most programs providing services for such children take a very different educational position concerning families. The literature provides a plethora of investigative studies stressing the effectiveness of the program and of the children when parents are working partners (Wiese, 1992; Breiner & Beck, 1984; Medway, 1989; Moreland, Schwebel, Beck, & Wells, 1982; Palmer & Cochran, 1988; Wiese & Kramer, 1988). Some of the issues discussed in this chapter are similar to the issues presented in Chapters 2 and 4. The perspective of this chapter is, however, completely different; the focus is on the need for and the how to's of parent education.

Parents who have been trained and educated to work with children at home provide a very important service and function to the educational system. Clearly, most educators do not have the time or the inclination to visit homes and work with children outside of the school setting. Without a doubt, the home has been described as the most natural of communication settings, given the everyday dynamics, daily activities, and family routines; but the educational system is not presently structured to provide services in the home. Therefore, the best alternative—and the one that appears to be most reasonable—is to train parents to work with children in a setting that is not available to the professional staff on an ongoing basis.

It is also the case that parents have "attitudes" concerning teachers and schools. They are suspicious because they do not understand and are not part of the daily activities of the child with disabilities. By educating parents and bringing them into the school, many of these attitudes can be changed. Parents learn about teachers and the educational process; they become part of the system. When parents are given a role in the education of their children, the home is brought to school and the school is brought home. There are two primary issues in the training process. The first issue involves *how* to teach parents procedurally to function as facilitators. What are the methods? What are some of the techniques that are presently being used? How are schools set up methodologically to train parents? The second issue involves *what* to teach parents—clearly more of a content-based factor. Do we teach them about child development? Do we teach them about language and cognition? Should this be an academically based program for parents that simulates what undergraduate and graduate students learn in their courses? How much information do we give to parents and on what topics? In considering these questions, it is obvious that we need to define more clearly what we want parents to *do* with their disabled children.

FAMILY INVOLVEMENT

In 1975, when Congress passed Public Law 94-142, the Education of All Handicapped Children Act, parental participation was stressed. The role of parents in the education of their children has been stressed in literature for disabled and nondisabled learners. In early intervention programs for preschool children, the teacher-parent relationship is critical in developing the parent-child relationship. One of the reasons that early intervention programs are so successful is the fact that the parents are acknowledged as primary teachers and facilitators of the children. If the parents are invested in their children's success, they will be committed to the educational process.

The parents provide a mechanism for generalization learning from the school setting to the home setting. There are a number of important factors that highlight the significance of the school-home relationship.

1. Early intervention programs for preschool children reflect the diversity of the community, and many programs exist in multicultural communities. As a result, preschool early intervention programs need to reflect and to address the diversity of family backgrounds. An important aspect of family intervention must be helping families acknowledge and accept the needs of the disabled child. Programs should provide families with a range of clinical support services in order to break through educational, attitudinal, social, and language barriers that interfere with child development and learning.

2. As discussed earlier, one way to change the role of the parent is to develop a more collaborative approach to decision making. Parents should be treated, recognized, and acknowledged as members of the child study team. Just as parents have access to reports and evaluations, they should also have access to the professional members of the team. Parents can contribute their insights, their experiences, and their knowledge of the child's problems and can also potentially extend educational learning to the home. For many parents, being a partner means being listened to and being respected. Clearly, educators need to incorporate the views of parents. A collaborative approach that allows parents to be part of the decision-making process would empower parents to become more actively involved in the educational process.

3. The starting point for parent education must be the parents' feelings and attitudes about the child. Schools need to develop a range of parent education services that address development, management, and feelings. If parents are going to be taught to manage their children effectively, they must receive formalized instruction. They must be encouraged to take on the responsibility of being facilitators. Schools must be encouraged to develop parent-training programs that would be effective in meeting the needs of multicultural families. Schools must be taught how to teach parents; parents in turn must be taught how to teach their children. Clearly, both will benefit from each other's contribution to the child.

4. In the process of incorporating parents and acknowledging their role, the structure and function of the school must change. Early intervention programs have a unique set of issues to address, one being that education cannot take place only in a classroom or only between the hours of 9:00 and 3:00. It must also take place at night and in the home. Early intervention programs must be flexible not only in their programming but also in terms of including other caregivers—siblings, grandparents, and baby-sitters. The educational process must extend to include the entire family, since it is really family empowerment that education is attempting to achieve. The more facilitators involved with the disabled preschooler, the greater the opportunity for language generalization. Each member of the family has something to contribute to the child; the school must have the flexibility to support each member's contribution.

5. Public Law 99-457 not only describes parental participation, but also focuses on the need for family intervention, as well as a family service plan (IFSP: Individual Family Service Program). Public Law 99-457 much more directly supports the role of the family in the intervention of the preschool child with disabilities. The IFSP details not only the needs of the child in early intervention programming but also specific services that the family can receive independent of the child.

The Family Constellation

In broadening our concept of the family, the notion of the traditional family is replaced by a family of caregivers. The preschool program is one of the initial agencies addressing the needs of families who are told for the first time that the child is disabled. There is obviously a tremendous amount of disillusionment and pain in the family as each individual grapples with the meaning and significance of the disability. Turnbull and Turnbull (1986) indicate that families must be prepared and strengthened to meet the needs of long-term issues with preschool children with language disorders. Early intervention provides the first step.

Parents must come to terms with the possibility that the preschool language-disordered child may one day be a disabled adult; long-term accommodations in the family must be acknowledged and addressed. If the traditional family demands that childrearing is basically the responsibility of the mother, the stress may be overwhelming. With each member of the family contributing supportively to the child and to each other, long-term problems are more readily and easily addressed. This is where the educational issues may be in conflict with cultural issues. It is important for the educational program to understand the cultural backgrounds of families in order to adequately reorganize family members to support each other in this lifelong process. The parents' cultural values will play a role in the development of strategies; an understanding of these values will facilitate the process of educational integration of the child in the family and the family in the school. Parents must be encouraged to participate and be involved in the child's educational development.

The Parent Partnership

Perhaps the most important aspect of this new relationship between the school and the home is the development of trust. Parents should have access to all reports, written materials, and evaluations of the child as well as frequent access to the classroom to view the child. Very often parents feel much more comfortable about separating from their three-year-olds when a teacher or social worker or psychologist is accessible on a regular basis. If parents have problems understanding technical reports and evaluations, a member of the professional team should be available to answer questions concerning the child's educational program. In addition, parents should feel that someone will get back to them quickly if there is a concern or a question. They should be assigned a specific professional, maybe the school psychologist or nurse, whom they can call whenever there is a family- or child-based problem. This "buddy" system between parents and professionals allows for the development of a trust-based relationship between the individuals who will work together for the benefit of the family and the program.

Parents should be included as part of the child's study team, which should meet on a monthly basis. They should be brought into these meetings to share their insights and knowledge, as well as to listen to the input from professionals. The educational goals for the child should be mutually agreed upon and mutually generated. Face-to-face discussions and personal interactions with the family are much more effective and trust building than formal letters and notes. Parents need to be kept informed of ongoing issues in the classroom, educational changes in the program, and curricula activities (Fitzgerald & Fischer, 1987).

For the most part, parents are not professionals and may be easily overwhelmed by technical reports and professional jargon. It is important for the professional members of the collaborative team to provide information that will be meaningful and relevant to the family. The professionals should not be condescending in their approach, but the information must be regulated, simplified, or modified so that parents can understand the technical terms. The more information that parents have access to, and the more they understand, the better equipped they will be to generalize their knowledge to the child in the home. It is to the benefit of both the school and the family for parents to visit the educational setting as much as possible. Sometimes technical reports are much more readily understood when children are viewed in terms of their peers, their teachers, and their learning activities.

Rogers-Warren and Warren (1983) discuss the fact that with the increasing demands on parents, there may be a detrimental side effect on family interactions. The introduction of a language/communication-disordered child presents a stress factor that may relate to the parents' feeling of isolation, responsibility, and blame. If they learn to share their concerns and feelings with educators, they will not feel so isolated and so responsible for the preschool child with a disability; the responsibility will be shared. Clearly, as early intervention expands in American education, educators must develop and explore the role of the parent as a primary contributor (Turnbull & Turnbull, 1982).

The language-disordered preschool child presents a constellation of problems to education. Because he or she must be viewed as a member of a family, it is the family that must be educated, facilitated, and supported. Early intervention, parent education, respite services, therapeutic services, and counseling services underscore the magnitude of a broad-based comprehensive approach to family involvement (Fitzgerald & Fischer, 1987). Education needs to develop a life-cycle continuum of services. Part of the parent-education experience is learning to understand the road ahead for the child who is disabled. It is far better to face, to discuss, and to address issues that may occur in the child's future than to deny the realities of the disabling problem.

Finally, as the field of child language development has changed to include pragmatic theories, the role of the family has been stressed. The preschool child with a language disorder must be viewed as a member of a family system. The communication that occurs within the family directly affects the child's language development. Parents, siblings, and extended family members all participate in a range of family-based experiences that highlight the uniqueness of each family system. Just as no two preschool children are the same, no two family systems are the same. In understanding the needs of the child, the professional must understand the family as an ecological system. The family provides a communication network, a communication environment in which the disabled child is affected by other family members. Educational goals in the classroom must reflect a sensitivity to family-based issues. The educational curriculum must target behaviors that will be generalized with the family system—within the family network.

Programmatic Issues

Given the available information on learning differences in the environment of children with and without disabilities and the fact that such input differences can interfere with language acquisition, form and content issues must be considered in parent programming. Specifically, *how* and *what* should professionals train parents of disabled children to do? This raises questions concerning methodological approaches to parent training. Several researchers have developed and implemented various caregiver training models.

Harris (1984) notes that as the perception of the nature of language disorders has changed from environmental to physiological, the role of parents in the treatment process has also changed. They are now recognized as integral members of the intervention team. The problem, however, involves the content of didactic parent training. The author noted that the *content* of parent-training programs reflects either a behavioral approach that ignores the broader family dynamics or a nonbehavioral approach that ignores didactic parent training. Harris proposes that effective treatment of the child involves an understanding of long-term changes and needs of the child's family. Family therapy, with its ecological focus, provides a more holistic approach to the child's growth and development. The family and its organizational structure provide the framework for understanding the child's potential for growth and development. The child with a disability needs the family to negotiate the environment for him or her. Harris describes that one year after the completion of a successful parent-training program, parents had discontinued use of the procedures they had been taught because of "lack of time, the child's limited ability to learn, the parents' perceived limits as teachers, and lack of professional support."

Behavioral management is not the only problem that families face. As the child with the disability grows up there are internal family issues that clearly affect him or her but are rarely addressed by professionals—marital stress, sibling problems, financial problems. These problems negatively influence the family's integrity and its ability to integrate the disabled child in its framework. When a family fights for its own survival, the child becomes another source of stress; he or she has the greatest opportunity to be nurtured in a family that has developed a sense of self-determination. No single individual or parent can maintain the sole responsibility for the disabled child's growth and development.

A behavioral technology that reflects the procedural aspects of how to teach is only part of the parent-training curriculum. Parents must be taught *what* to teach—the content of the instruction to their children (Fox & Westling, 1991). Families need to understand that the developmental stages in their child are delayed and that their expectations must be altered. In addition, because parents of a language/communication-disordered child are deprived of the experiences that follow the normal stages of development and reflect a child's developing independence, they need to come to terms with the fact that they will not always be around to take care of their child as he or she grows to adulthood. Intervention needs to expand beyond behavioral technology to include family issues, emotional aspects, and dynamics of family members and stages of family development.

McDade and Varnedoe (1987) note that one of the most difficult issues in developing a program for parents relates to *who* the client is. They suggest that in a parent-training program, the parent must be the client and the success of the program relates specifically to how effectively parents' interactive behaviors are changed. This becomes a difficult issue for schools and clinics that provide services directly to children. As the severity of the child's problem becomes more of a critical variable in the child's prognosis, the more important becomes the role of parents and caregivers. With a severely involved child, the disability requires a level of therapeutic intervention that cannot be limited to a center, a school, a therapist, or a specific set of half hours during the course of the week.

In the last analysis, the multiple services can be fragmenting for the child because they are not integrated into other areas of life, particularly the home. The parents, who are the only consistent individuals from setting to setting and time to time, often do not receive direct instruction in educational programs and therapeutic contexts (Cartright & Ruscello, 1979).

McDade and Varnedoe (1987) discuss several variables that should be included in the content of a parent-education program. Language facilitative techniques include training parents to provide positive feedback for children's communicative attempts. This stresses the importance of communication and de-emphasizes the attention parents often pay to structural and syntactic aspects of their children's speech. Parents are also taught to use expansions and comments to facilitate children's language. In this parent-training program parents are trained individually during thirty-minute weekly sessions for eight to ten weeks. Parent-child dyadic interactions are videotaped to determine initial parent-training goals. Parents are dismissed from parent training once they demonstrate that they can exhibit a set of target behaviors. The researchers noted that there are limitations in the use of video equipment that involve additional time and space.

Fitzgerald and Karnes (1987) describe the RIP (Regional Intervention Programs for Parents and Preschools) service delivery system, which has been used in the treatment of families with young at-risk children with developmental disabilities. Parental involvement is central to the RIP model (Timm & Rule, 1981). Parents function as change agents, as case managers for other parents, and as evaluators of the program's success. Parental participation has two operational phases—a treatment phase and a generalization phase. In the treatment phase, parents work individually with their own children at home and at the RIP site. When this phase has been completed, they give their time and skills to train other, newer parents, conduct interviews, collect and analyze data, and teach in the classroom. The RIP model uses trained parents as the cornerstone of the operation of the program, effectively addressing the problem of generalization of skills to other contexts and agents. The level of involvement of parents is both an advantage and a disadvantage. Although the success of the program relates to the role of the parents, there are many parents who do not want to be taught by other parents nor do they want the responsibilities of teaching their own children.

Fitzgerald and Fischer (1987) describe the Mama Lere parent-infant training program, which has four service delivery components: supportive counseling, educational advocacy, information exchange, and communicative facilitation. The program is based on an ecological model that stresses the fact that only families can provide long-term support and commitment to the child with a disability. In facilitating the development of the child, the unique needs of the family must be translated into programmatic information. Parents have a number of programming options. Families can actually choose the type of service they prefer—an individual format with professional staff members, group discussions with other families, or individual discussions with families who share a common problem. Parents are provided with developmental information in all areas of instruction and are encouraged to express their perceptions and concerns in discussion groups. Information instruction is a primary factor in the family-based habilitation process. Another important component is the notion that parental advocacy is a positive process involving knowledge, rights, and responsibilities. Advocacy training involves an understanding of educational procedures and options as well as political possibilities in the event of educational dispute. With advocacy comes the family's realization that parents must never give up their decision making. Ultimately, with advocacy comes self-determination.

THE SCHOOL FOR LANGUAGE AND COMMUNICATION DEVELOPMENT

In the remainder of this chapter, the parent-training program that has been developed and utilized at SLCD for the past eight years will be presented and discussed. The training program is based on the belief (emphasized in the research literature over the past ten years) that the role of the parent as a partner is critical in the educational process of the preschool child with a language disorder. SLCD's extensive program has been evaluated annually through grant projects; it is described here as a possible model for students and educators interested in understanding and analyzing a working program.

At SLCD the parent is recognized as a language facilitator. Several studies have reevaluated the role of the parent in terms of the input provided in the developmental process (Snow, Midkiff-Borunda, Small, & Proctor, 1984; Cross, 1977; Lieven, 1984; Tiegerman & Siperstein, 1984). These investigations suggest that the parents' input stresses the highly individualized relationships between parent and child. In the communication process, it has been noted that there is a breakdown in the communication interaction between parents and language-disordered children (Tiegerman & Siperstein, 1982, 1984). This literature suggests that parents of a child with a language disorder are at a serious disadvantage because the communication process is not reciprocal in nature. They do not know how to facilitate development in their child; they do the best they can, but they are often frustrated. Parents must be trained to regulate the form and content of their own language in order to stimulate children's language growth. Obviously, to do this, parents must know about form and content issues.

At the School for Language and Communication Development, parents are provided with a number of parent-training experiences that enable them to understand the educational goals in the classroom. First, they have an opportunity to observe their children in a language-learning group—the classroom. Second, they participate in a formal language-training seminar, which serves many purposes. As a prerequisite to working with their children, parents need a theoretical foundation. The parent-training seminar ties in with observation of the classroom and of therapeutic services. Parents have the opportunity to look at the classroom while theoretical and procedural materials are discussed in the seminar. Once a theoretical framework is established, they can be shown how to apply their knowledge at home with their children. The extensive programming reinforces the idea that they play a primary role in the language facilitation of the child. To adequately perform this function, they proceed through a program with the following components:

1. parent as student;
2. parent as observer;
3. parent as child facilitator;
4. parent as assistant;
5. parent as advocate;
6. parent as parent facilitator.

Parent as Student

Parent-education classes provide an excellent forum for teaching parents about developmental disabilities and educational decision making (McDade & Simpson, 1984; Kaiser, Fischer, Alpert, Hemmeter, Tiernan, & Ostrosky, 1990). The topics presented in the classes range in diversity from normal developmental issues to management techniques to IFSP goals. Figure 6-1 shows that when presented with the opportunity to attend instructional classes, parents become actively involved. Such classes provide definitions of technical terms, so that parents can more competently contribute to educational exchange and more adequately understand reports and evaluations. Classes can also provide developmental charts and materials so that parents can understand their child's level of functioning in relation to the normal developmental sequence. Professionals from different disciplines (psychology, reading, occupational therapy, etc.) can lecture on educational goals and therapeutic instructional techniques. Parents can learn about the educational process, philosophy, and integration of related services and can be taught *how* to work with their children at home. Specifically, the procedural techniques that are used with parents can facilitate child changes achieved in school.

The development of parents' academic knowledge should be very similar to the development of knowledge in a professional. At no time should parents be made to feel that the material is being "watered down" or that there is an expectation that they will not utilize this knowledge. The intent and motivation of professionals should be very clear—that parents must understand that if they are going to function effectively with their children they are going to have to *know* what to do. These classes can require readings, simple examinations,

Figure 6-1
Should Parents Be Educated to Work with Their Children? How?

. . . Yes, though parent-training classes.

. . . First, a parent has to be aware of the problem. Second, constant communication between parent and teachers is important.

. . . Yes. In my case I read a lot about language development and try to utilize the knowledge.

. . . A parent can become educated by reading information on the disabling condition, going to meetings and rap sessions. Discussing feelings and concerns with others with the same problems and professionals are a great help.

. . . Yes, by taking the school work and reinforcing what the child has learned. Especially from their individual speech teacher.

. . . Yes, programs that provide parent training should focus on reinforcing the learning that takes place in the classroom.

. . . Through workshops, literature, and advice from teachers.

. . . Yes, they should be told to participate with the child. It should be a requirement.

. . . Every parent has to find their own way of dealing with it. I joined by local SEPTA and volunteered as a parent member, learning the laws and rights of children with disabilities.

. . . Join groups—speak to parents that have children with similar problems.

. . . At best, parents should seek to become educated and realize that the learning process is always ongoing. Providers of services to children are in the best position to offer support services to parents.

. . . Yes, having a "special" child means adapting to your child's special needs. Parent-training classes at SLCD provide parents with an understanding of their child's needs, problems, and modes of treatment. This helps facilitate communication more effectively.

. . . The answer is yes. And the *how* is easy, it is the time that is required to get the education.

and parent contributions. Perhaps even parent lectures would be helpful in getting parents to utilize their knowledge in class with other parents. This is an excellent exercise, since eventually the parents will have to be able to express themselves as contributing members of multidisciplinary teams. Parents who present themselves at district multidisciplinary meetings as sophisticated and knowledgeable are taken quite seriously by the professional team.

Academic knowledge concerning child language development and an understanding of the educational process are invaluable to the parents of language- and communication-disordered children not only in terms of a short-term experience but also in terms of long-term advocacy. Basically, it is the parents who live with the child. They have experiences in the home that professionals cannot possibly understand. Ultimately, the parents remain with the child and advocate for the child while professionals come and go in the child's life. The parents provide the consistency and the continuity that the professional community can never provide.

In order for parents to ultimately function as facilitators and teachers, they must first be students (Bruder & Bricker, 1985). In the framework of the classroom, they can be taught many of the skills involved in education development and facilitation. The primary assumption is that the parents' interactive behavior with the child must be changed. In changing the nature and structure of the adults' input to the child, the child's language will be facilitated and will, therefore, change. McDade and Varnedoe (1987) indicate that in training parents to function as intervention agents for the language-disordered child, there is an implicit acknowledgment, specifically "that someone else is capable of functioning in the child's behalf as a primary agent."

When parents receive educational instruction, the child's language training is expanded and broadened. Because the parents are taught as students, they acquire a unique understanding of what the child is progressing through, since he or she is *also* a student. Classroom instruction for parents involves teaching them *how* to teach—how to facilitate interactive language behavior in the disordered child. They learn about being agents of change; they learn what must be changed in the child's home environment. They become sensitively attuned to the child's language behaviors and begin to see themselves as significant factors in the development of their children. By treating parents as students, the program formalizes the educational process with the family and brings the family into the school environment. It is obvious that as part of this programming a curriculum for parent education must be developed, implemented, and evaluated over time (Fitzgerald & Karnes, 1987). Success in such a curriculum will obviously be a function of many different variables.

Cultural Background

One of the most complex problems facing education is the diversity of cultures that are represented in many schools. The educational system must take into consideration various backgrounds of parents and families. Obviously, cultural differences will affect the parent-education process. Parents will present different attitudes, different concerns, and different biases about the disordered child, education, and their role as facilitators.

Educational Level

Parents with extensive educational training have the ability to integrate information more quickly and actualize on what they have learned in training classes for their child. Parents' educational background, level, and discipline will affect the nature of the interaction between the school educator and the parent. The content of programming, as well as the extent of training, will be affected by parents' educational background. The parent who has not graduated from high school obviously will require a great deal more direction and support and intervention than the parent who is a teacher.

Economic Level

The financial factors that affect the family will also affect the child. The single-parent family requires special training and intervention. Single parents who must work to support their families are already stressed by social, economic, familial, and child-based issues. They will be difficult to reach during the day. It will be difficult for them to attend parent-education classes during the day. The educational system must make a commitment to nontraditional families and provide alternative training sessions on weekends and in the evening. The single mother who is struggling to support her children must give priority to her job. Teachers must learn to take into account the factors that affect the ecological health and welfare of the family.

Involvement with the Child

Traditionally, mothers have been much more involved in the rearing and nurturance of young children. The preschool child with a severe language disorder presents a significant stress on family dynamics and interactions. Very often fathers take the position that managing the child is "Mommy's job." In the traditional situation where fathers tend not to be involved, the presence of the disabled child makes it even more difficult for the father to assume responsibilities when the mother is not around. Fathers have different issues than mothers as far as children are concerned. Training classes for fathers obviously must also be offered at alternate times—on weekends and in the evening—and the content of programming may also be different for fathers. Figure 6-2 describes some of the differing attitudes that mothers and fathers present at the beginning of parent training. The more parents work together in supporting each other and working with the child, the greater the opportunity will be for the family to function as a unit and for each adult to provide respite for the

Figure 6-2
Mothers' and Fathers' Attitudes

Mothers

1. I feel totally overwhelmed with my disabled child.
2. I do not have any time to spend with my other children or my husband.
3. I do not have any time for myself, and I am stressed out.
4. My husband feels that along with housekeeping, washing, cleaning, and disciplining, my disabled child is my problem and responsibility.
5. I am very concerned that my husband is afraid of our disabled child.

Fathers

1. I work. That is my primary responsibility. My wife takes care of the kids.
2. I try to help my wife, but she is much more effective in managing our disabled son.
3. My son with disabilities listens to his mother more than he listens to me.
4. After working all day I really don't want to be bothered with the noisy havoc in the house.
5. I cannot go to work in the morning with all the craziness that goes on. I cannot stand the confusion, the screaming, and the mess.

other. Time together and time alone are very important issues in any family but they are especially important in a family that includes a preschool child with a language disorder.

The Effectiveness of Instruction

Over time, parent education and programming will change. The program should be evaluated annually; Figure 6-3 provides an example of a questionnaire to be filled out by parents who have been through the program. (Programs are only as effective as the parents who participate in them.) At the end of the year short-term and long-term analyses are helpful in providing a feedback mechanism to fine-tune procedures and content.

Parent training will be changed many times over the course of the school year. In individualizing the parent-instruction process, the specific needs of the parent and the family can be addressed by evaluating the curricula on an ongoing basis. As students, parents at SLCD attend two one-hour weekly classes dealing with the following topics: normal language and communication development, communication disorders, communication intervention programming, social development, social interaction, play development, and specialty topics. They are presented with a reading list and trained to analyze adult-child interactions from videotapes (see the section on Parent as Child Facilitator and Figure 6-4).

Parent as Observer

Parents are required to participate in the classroom with their children on a weekly basis. The teachers provide the appropriate models for interaction and parents have an opportunity to observe the instructional activities that set the occasion for social communication. They learn how to interact with their children in ways that facilitate communication. They can also observe the classroom by means of a closed-circuit video system. This nonintrusive mechanism allows them to watch the child in all of the specialty therapies and learning contexts without interfering in the instruction. Parents often comment on how many different things they see in their children when they are not around (see Figure 6-5).

Parent as Child Facilitator

Parents are videotaped during play interactions with their children (Moran & Whitman, 1985), and the videotapes are analyzed to determine the forms and communicative aspects of the adult-child interaction. The form displayed in Figure 6-4, which is used to transcribe parent-child conversational utterances, also allows the parents to categorize the semantic function of the linguistic input provided to the child. They can also determine the number of communicative turns that occur on each topic—the greater the number of turns, the more sophisticated the child's language abilities. Parents can also assess semantic

Figure 6-3
Parent Attitudinal Scale

Please circle: Male

Female

Please fill out the following questionnaire. Rate your responses according to the following:

1	2	3	4	5
Strongly Agree (SA)	Agree (A)	Don't Know (?)	Disagree (D)	Strongly Disagree (SD)

	SA	A	?	D	SD
Questions	**1**	**2**	**3**	**4**	**5**
1. My child's problem is so serious I can't deal.					
2. My child is unmanageable.					
3. I'm a better manager than my spouse.					
4. I don't like that my child has behavior problems.					
5. I'm embarrassed by my child's behavior problems.					
6. I would describe my child's behavior problem as serious.					
7. I'm embarrassed my child has a disabling condition.					
8. My family does not understand my child's behavior problems.					
9. I don't understand why my child acts out.					
10. I feel I did something wrong.					
11. My other children don't understand why my child acts out.					
12. Having a disabled child is very difficult.					
13. I like to interact with child.					
14. My child is difficult to interact with.					
15. My child is not normal, so I do not talk to him/her the same as another child.					
16. My child acts out all the time.					
17. I can only manage my child by being physical.					
18. I can only manage my child by yelling.					
19. I can only manage my child by putting him/her in his/her room.					
20. My child cannot play with other children.					

Figure 6-3
Continued

	SA	A	?	D	SD
Questions	**1**	**2**	**3**	**4**	**5**
21. I am frustrated managing my child.					
22. I wish my child would listen.					
23. In managing my disabled child, the other siblings are ignored.					
24. My spouse and I argue about how to manage our disabled child.					
25. There is conflict between my spouse and me because we have a disabled child.					
26. If my child were normal, my spouse and I would interact more with our disabled child.					
27. My spouse leaves the managing of our child to me.					
28. I would like to know how to manage my child more successfully.					
29. This course has taught me how to manage my child's problem.					
30. I feel better about myself.					
31. I understand my child's needs better.					
32. I understand what it means to be language disordered.					
33. I understand that as language increases, behavior improves.					
34. I think every parent needs to take a parent training course.					
35. Parent education is just as important as my child's education.					
36. This parent training class has improved my relationship with my other children.					
37. This parent training class has improved my relationship with my spouse.					
38. Parent training has improved my self-confidence.					
39. I am willing to change my behavior to meet my child's needs.					
40. I know how to change my behavior to meet my child's needs.					
41. Having a disabled child is a learning process.					

Figure 6-3
Continued

Questions	SA 1	A 2	? 3	D 4	SD 5
42. The Committee on Preschool Special Education (CPSE) process is difficult.					
43. I am aware of all the rights, rules, procedures, and regulations regarding my child's education.					
44. I feel I can adequately advocate for my child's needs.					
45. I accept my role in the CPSE process.					
46. I accept my role in the placement decisions of my child's education.					
47. I have the power to make educational decisions related to my child.					
48. I am comfortable with the role I have in my child's education.					
49. My disabled child needs more attention than a nondisabled child.					
50. My child's teachers and school are responsible for providing me with the information I need about my child's needs and rights.					
51. I am responsible for learning what my child's needs and rights are.					
Comments:					

knowledge by analyzing the child's descriptive detail on each topic. Based on the analysis, parents are provided with prescriptive training on how to facilitate communicative interaction given the nature of their children's language-learning needs. They are trained to transcribe and analyze language samples as a means of monitoring ongoing adult-child communication and language changes in class and at home. Adult-child videotapes are used for parent-training and parent-child assessment purposes.

Parent as Assistant

During the latter half of the training year, parents are gradually integrated into the classroom context, providing them with the opportunity to interact and apply their classroom

Figure 6-4
Semantic Relatedness

Type of Session: Child Number: Page:

Type of Number: Parent Name:

Context:			Semantic Category
Verbal	Child	Adult	
Nonverbal			

Context:			Semantic Category
Verbal	Child	Adult	
Nonverbal			

Context:			Semantic Category
Verbal	Child	Adult	
Nonverbal			

Context:			Semantic Category
Verbal	Child	Adult	
Nonverbal			

Figure 6-5
Parental Observations

1. I was surprised to see how my child interacted with other children.
2. Since my child always had temper tantrums at home, I was amazed to see how responsive he was to his teacher's directions.
3. In observing my child in his classroom, I had the opportunity to watch the teacher use specific procedures and techniques.
4. I had never seen my child function in a group situation. Watching him with other children gave me a whole different picture.
5. I never saw my child bite another child before.
6. I never saw how my child became frustrated in a large social group.
7. I never saw how my child interacted nonverbally with other children.

knowledge under the direct supervision of the teaching staff. This also stimulates generalized learning to the home situation (Moran & Whitman, 1985; Mahoney & Powell, 1988).

Parent as Advocate

The process of becoming partners in the educational process encourages parents to become more assertive and more independent (Schaefer, 1989; Parks & Smeriglio, 1986). This is a challenge to the educational system and to professionals. As parents become more sophisticated, they naturally become more involved and more demanding in terms of decision making. The educational system cannot do it all from 9:00 A.M. to 3:00 P.M. Parents are a resource; they must be educated to function in the system. Part of the challenge of involvement is advocacy (Healy, Keesee, & Smith, 1989).

Sophisticated and knowledgeable parents question. They challenge the decisions of professionals, multidisciplinary teams, and Committees on Preschool Special Education. They can advocate for their children's needs in a way that no professional team ever can. Parents have an investment in their children and their growth, short-term and long-term. One of the issues in education involves an understanding of educational policy, legislation, and law. Part of the parent-training experience should be devoted specifically to advocacy issues so that parents do not step into team meetings without a firm understanding of process, procedure, and protocol.

Parents who understand their role know what to expect and how to contribute effectively to the decision-making process of the educational team (Yell & Espin, 1990). Parents who "know" about their children can understand their needs, can explain IFSP goals, and can contribute to team decision making. It is important to understand that professionals see the child for a limited amount of time in a rather artificial setting, whereas parents can present a set of long-term observations and issues. Early intervention programs can have a long-term impact on parent education by including advocacy training. A gift for a parent of a preschool child is the ability to advocate for the child's needs as he or she gets older and enters school-age programming. Early intervention programs can begin the process by training parents to function effectively as advocates for their children.

Parent as Parent Facilitator

For parents who have been through the academic experience of training classes, parent networking provides a form of validation for other parents of language- and communication-disordered children. There are things that parents can say to other parents that professionals can never say. One forum for parent networking is a twelve-step program that is run as a group experience by parents for parents entering the special education system. The purpose of the step program is to allow parents to share their fears and frustrations with other parents who have been through the system and who are further along the life-cycle process (National Center for Family-Centered Care, 1990).

The step program allows parents to learn through sharing—to learn that their feelings, fears, frustrations, and expectations are understandable. Through the sharing process parents learn to come to terms with the life cycle and accept the child as an individual separate and whole. The step program respects anonymity and the confidentiality of families and their issues. Step programs can be developed by parents based on other step formats; the group exchange process has been extremely successful with other groups of individuals attempting to grapple with serious social and family issues. Parents need to feel that they are not alone, that there is a networking system for families and parents who have been through similar experiences. They need to have a place to share their fears and their feelings. The step program also infuses a sense of empowerment and responsibility not only to one's own family but to other families who are going through a similar experience; sharing is healing. Parents helping parents provides a lifeline and a continuum for learning about personal responsibility.

CONTENT ISSUES IN PARENT TRAINING

One of the issues noted in the introduction to this section was the fact that there are two significant components in a parent-education program. The content of parent instruction involves the substance of knowledge provided to families. What should parents know? What should parents learn to do with the language-disordered child? As part of the generalization process between school-based knowledge and home-based instruction, it is important to give parents the same knowledge base that the teacher received in her academic training program. If teachers and parents share the same knowledge base, philosophy, and procedures, the generalization process has a greater opportunity for success in integrating the school and the home. The parent clearly is the liaison between the classroom and the home environment (Hess & Holloway, 1984).

Semantic Approach

A semantic learning approach teaches parents to analyze their interactions with the language-disordered child and to be semantically related to the child's language-learning experience. Snow and Ferguson (1977) provide the basis for the content aspect of programming. Semantic relatedness deals with maternal language. Maternal input must be child-sensitive and contextually based. This interactional model proposes that adult input can provide a significant source of learning for the child. In fact, the term *motherese* was coined to describe the language produced by a mother when she regulates and attunes herself to her child's language-learning needs.

The interaction between mother and child is similar to the language lesson that might occur between a teacher and a child. The activities that occur at home in daily living are a primary source of language learning. Maternal regulation is the result of social interaction and tends to be child-focused, child-centered, and child-oriented. Maternal input serves to enhance the child's acquisition of language by providing a framework for learning.

In being semantically related, the mother's input is directly a function of what the child is doing and saying in the immediate context. Mother stays on topic and follows the child in terms of his verbalizations and actions. Mother talks about the context in which the child is involved. The child's actions are the focus of her attention. Mother expands on what the child says, provides additional information, and naturally ties together the relationship between what he is doing and "how you describe what is happening." Snow and Ferguson (1977) noted that approximately 70 percent of mother's input is directly related to the child's vocal, verbal, and nonverbal behavior.

Structure and Relatedness

Mothers are also taught that it is important to pay attention to the child's linguistic abilities and to regulate their language structure to the child's level of comprehension. Maternal utterances, therefore, are short and simple. They may consist of a single clause, but they provide a basic structural model for the child. As the linguistic structure of the child's language becomes more sophisticated, mother increases the syntactic complexity of her model.

Mothers are taught to use the daily routines of dressing, washing, eating, and playing as language lessons. Establishing routines at home, talking about those routines, and breaking routines so that there are unanticipated consequences are important aspects of language lessons in the home environment. Other members of the family, grandparents, and siblings are also brought into the language lesson. In extending the language-learning experience into the home environment, the opportunity for generalization increases.

Semantic Categories and Contingencies

During the first fifteen weeks of the class, parents are given specific training in categories of semantic relatedness. Figure 6-6 presents the training categories and the definitions for each semantic category. One semantic category is presented each week. The past weeks' categories are reviewed by means of a homework assignment. Each week the parent is given a worksheet that must be completed during a play activity with the child. During a nonstructured play activity, the parent is asked to record the parent-child interaction (see Figure 6-4). This language analysis is submitted the following week to the speech/language pathologist teaching the class and analyzed by semantic category and by several other conversational language variables.

Figure 6-6
Coding Key and Category Definitions: Semantic Relatedness (Analysis I)

Code	Category Definition
RNVA	Maternal statement related to *child's nonverbal activity* (to what child is looking at, pointing to, action he/she is performing).
ERNVA*	Maternal *elicitation related to child's nonverbal activity* (question, statement whose purpose is to elicit verbal information from child).
NRNVA	Maternal utterances *not related* to child's nonverbal activity.
RNVV	Maternal utterance related to child's nonverbal vocalizations (these utterances include imitations, interpretation, and elicitations).
NRNVV	Maternal utterance *not related* to child's nonverbal vocalization.
Imit.	Maternal *imitations* related to child's utterance (imitations may be partial or complete).
Exp.	Maternal *expansion* of the child's utterance (filling in omitted function words and grammatical markers).
Ext.	Maternal extension of the child's utterance (new information and grammatical markers are added).
Elicit.	Maternal *elicitation* of words related to child's utterance (questions and/or statements).
Other	Maternal utterances related to child's verbal activity that are acknowledgements (e.g., "ok," "very good," "yes").
NRVA	Maternal utterances *not related* to child's verbal activity (previous utterance).
NC*	*Nonclassifiable*—maternal and/or child statements that are *unintelligible*.
NS*	*Nonscorable*—any disagreement in coding a particular nonverbal/verbal interaction.

*Additional categories not utilized by Snow (1979).

Figure 6-7
Topic Maintenance/Dyadic Interaction (Analysis II)

Code	Category Definition
S	*Speaker-Initiator*—speaker who acts as initiator of topic of conversation
R	*Speaker-Responder*—speaker who responds to previous statement during topic of conversation.
NR	*No response* to a Speaker-Initiator/Speaker-Responder
I	*Inappropriate*—statement made a S or R, inappropriate to topic established.
V	*Verbal*
NV	*Nonverbal*
NC	*Nonclassifiable*
NS	*Nonscorable*

The parent language-training component shown in Figure 6-7 consists of formalized child-language measures. Parents are taught to utilize each of the semantic categories and are required to do a language sample on a weekly basis. This aspect of the training program was designed with the following goals in mind:

1. In order to determine the parent-child language interaction, semantic categories are discussed and then measured. The language analysis of the mother-child interaction serves to identify communication differences that interfere with the dyadic exchange process. This provides an analysis of the language-learning needs of the child, not only as an individual language user but in a communicative social framework (McLean & Vincent, 1984).
2. In order to reinforce language development at home, parents are trained to facilitate language. The generalization process provides further information for stimulation of child-language development since parents are actively involved in language-based activities.
3. The content of the programming focuses the parents' attention on specific language-learning variables in the child. Parents can be trained to regulate the complexity of their input along with the content of their language. This provides the child with highly specialized input in school as well as at home.
4. Requiring that parents engage in a weekly language sample allows for self-evaluation and feedback. Parents can analyze on paper the relationship between the semantic categories presented and the child's language responses. Regulating the parents' language behavior results in observable and measurable changes in child language behavior (Cordisco & Strain, 1986).

After the semantic contingency training has been completed, parents are provided with formal instruction on language development components. The

Bloom and Lahey model is presented and each area of language development is discussed: pragmatic, semantic, syntactic, and metalinguistic. Parents are provided with definitions, worksheets, home-based activities, and homework assignments. The curriculum used in introductory language-development courses for undergraduate students is utilized with the same degree of detail for parents in the training class. Parents are given midterm and final exams. If they pass the final, they go to an advanced training course. If they do not, they are required to repeat the training course at the introductory level.

PARENT EMPOWERMENT

Educational laws and policies have changed over the past several decades. Demands on schools and teachers given multicultural issues and programming for the disabled have altered educational priorities, programs, and procedures. Educational accomplishments have *not* been outstanding in the public schools; community issues are diverse and complex. Educational programming for the disabled has provided a great deal of information that can be generalized to nondisabled children and their families. Clearly, education cannot accomplish everything for everyone without the support and integration of families. The traditional family may have changed in its form and structure but its contribution to child development and education has not; parents and extended families represent an untapped resource for education.

Schools and programs need to refocus the educational process to incorporate the family. Viewing the child in the framework of the family is an important initial step. The entire philosophy of education must be changed. Education cannot be confined to 9:00 A.M. to 3:00 P.M.; it is an all-day, everyplace process for the language-disordered child. The schoolteacher cannot be the only facilitator and educator; family members must be trained and recruited to take on the role and the responsibility to extend the educational process into the home (McDade & Simpson, 1984). This clearly will ease the burden on an already overburdened school system.

In this extension process, schools and teachers will have to relinquish their control over many aspects of education. Parents will have to be trained to function as decision makers and contributors to the system. Training parents empowers them to contribute and to disagree, which presents a dilemma for most professionals. The benefits of actively involved parents will ultimately enrich the language-disordered child's opportunities for learning and success. As the role of the family changes, so too must the role of the teacher. Parents and professionals must learn a new collaborative relationship in decision making (Turnbull & Turnbull, 1986). Often there is great fear and risk related to change. To quote Toya Davis, "Given the problems in education, the system cannot afford *not* to change." She is right!

SUMMARY

This chapter has discussed the need for formalized parent education. It is important for the student of education to understand that education as a whole is going through many changes. The issues faced by parents of disabled children are real issues faced by *all* parents whose children attend school. The problems in the American family are very similar to problems faced by teachers in schools. It is critical to understand that today's student will be the teacher of tomorrow, who must face these changes and understand the history as well as the basis for parent empowerment and child advocacy. Let us look forward and view these changes as a positive movement; the realignment of parent and professional presents a great opportunity and potential for education. Let us look forward to a time when parents and professionals can share in the decision-making process; the ultimate investment is the product of both—the child.

A FEW WORDS FROM TOYA DAVIS

Chapter 6 discussed many issues related to parent training and education. I remember sitting in one of Dr. Tiegerman's earliest classes and shaking my head and thinking I could never do half of the things that she was talking about. Today I teach these parent and education classes and I function on Governor Cuomo's preschool advisory council. I feel strongly about the fact that education will only be successful when parents are involved in the instructional process. Parents need to know how to teach their children. Parents need to be taught so that they in turn can teach. I feel I have been very fortunate. I attended all of the parent education classes, observed my son on a weekly basis, and worked with him every day when he came home from school. I was treated as an equal and a partner in the educational process. I was welcomed into the classroom, but it was also clear to me that I had a responsibility to do my part. That is what is most interesting about the partnership in education. It does not mean that teachers and educators will be giving away their power. It means that we will share in our responsibilities toward the child.

It was amazing to me to watch Jonathan in class. There were so many things that I saw him do in school that did not occur at home. I saw him for the first time with other children. I saw him play. I heard him speak. I watched all of the activities. I watched the teacher and how she managed him. Then I could take all this information and talk about it in my parent-training class and generalize it to my home with my husband. I believe very strongly in parent education—not hand-holding, but education. There is nothing more important than to know about one's child. I can also help other parents. I can say things as a parent of a handicapped child that Dr. Tiegerman could never say. Having been taught, I can now teach. I see my role and my responsibility, and I encourage other parents to become part of the learning process.

As a parent of a handicapped child I feel I have learned a great deal about the educational process and about empowerment in the process. I feel that I have been very fortunate since the program that my Jonathan attended took the issue of parent training and advocacy seriously. The school viewed the parent as the primary facilitator in a child's life and as a result, they provided parent-education programs and peer support groups for mothers and fathers. I attended the parent-training classes with many other parents; classes were scheduled during the day and the evening so that parents with different work schedules could be accommodated.

The parent-education class was taught by Dr. Tiegerman and her professional staff. There was a structured curriculum that was similar to Dr. Tiegerman's graduate courses at the university in language development and language disorders. The academic lectures were combined with classroom observations since the school had a closed-circuit video system and a television camera in every classroom. I could learn about pragmatic communicative functions in the parent-training class and then observe how communication behaviors were facilitated in Jonathan's class. There were reading assignments, lectures, and examinations. I learned about what it meant to be language disordered as a child. I learned how to teach Jonathan at home and in contexts outside of school. I became one of Jonathan's teachers; I could actively participate in his growth and development. I felt invigorated, mobilized, and empowered by my new responsibility and role. Perhaps one of the greatest compliments that I ever received occurred after a conversation with the chairperson of my district's CSE. He asked me if I were a speech-language pathologist. I had learned to be a teacher and an advocate for Jonathan, skills that I could take with me as Jonathan progressed through his educational career. I knew that I could and would always be there for him as an active contributor. I feel that I have learned enough about the educational system and my son's learning difficulties that I can function as an effective advocate.

The educational system with all of its rules, regulations, and laws is very complicated. When parents enter the system they are initially overwhelmed by the fact that their child is handicapped. The fact that the system is so complicated is an additional burden for families entering the process. I believe that parents must be incorporated into the child's education. I believe that all parents should be trained and educated whether the child is in special education, regular education, or gifted programming. I have learned that as Jonathan's advocate, I can only function effectively if I know about my child and his learning problems. I can only contribute to his education if I know about educational procedures and techniques. I can only be a decision maker if I have enough knowledge to make a decision. I feel that educational programs and schools around the country should develop education classes for parents.

REFERENCES

Breiner, J., & Beck, S. (1984). Parents as change agents in the management of their developmentally delayed children's noncompliant behaviors: A critical review. *Applied Research in Mental Retardation, 5,* 259–278.

Bruder, M., & Bricker, D. (1985). Parents as teachers of their children and other parents. *Journal of the Division for Early Childhood, 9,* 136–150.

Cartright, L., & Ruscello, D. (1979). A survey of parent involvement practices in the speech clinic. *ASHA, 21,* 275–279.

Cordisco, L. K., & Strain, P. S. (1986). Assessment of generalization and maintenance in a multicomponent parent training program. *Journal of the Division for Early Childhood, 10,* 10–24.

Cross, T. (1977). Mothers' speech adjustments: The contribution of selected child listener variables. In C. Snow & C. Ferguson (Eds.), *Talking to children.* London: Cambridge University Press.

Fitzgerald, M. T., & Fischer, R. M. (1987, June). A family involvement model for hearing impaired infants. *Topics in Language Disorders.*

Fitzgerald, M. T., & Karnes, D. E. (1987, June). A parent-implemented language model for at risk and developmentally delayed preschool children. *Topics in Language Disorders.*

Fox, L., & Westling, D. (1991). A preliminary evaluation of training parents to use facilitative strategies with their children with profound disabilities. *JASH, 16,* 168–176.

Harris, S. L. (1984, January). The family and the autistic child: A behavioral perspective. *Family Relations.*

Healy, A., Keesee, P., & Smith, B. (1989). *Early services for children with special needs: Transactions for family support.* Iowa City: University Hospital School.

Hess, R. D., & Holloway, S. D. (1984). Family and school as educational institutions. In R. D. Parke, R. N. Emde, H. P. McAdoo, & G. P. Sackett (Eds.), *Review of child development research: Vol. 7* (pp. 179–222). Chicago: University of Chicago Press.

Kaiser, A. P., Fischer, R., Alpert, C. L., Hemmeter, M. L., Tiernan, M., & Ostrosky, M. (1990). Toward a hybrid model of parent-implemented language intervention: Analysis of the effects of milieu and responsive-interaction teaching by parents. Paper presented at the annual meeting of the American Association on Mental Retardation, Atlanta, GA.

Lieven, E. V. M. (1984). Intervention style and children's language learning. *Topics in Language Disorders, 4* (4), 15–23.

Mahoney, G., & Powell, G. (1988). Modifying parent-child interaction: Enhancing the development of handicapped children. *The Journal of Special Education, 22,* 82–96.

McDade, H., & Simpson, M. (1984). Use of instruction, modeling and videotape feedback to modify parent behavior. A strategy for facilitating language development in the home. *Seminars in Speech and Language, 5* (3), 229–240.

McDade, H., & Varnedoe, D. (1987). Training parents to be language facilitators. *Topics in Language Disorders, 7,* 19–30.

McLean, M., & Vincent, L. (1984). The use of expansions as language intervention technique in the natural environment. *Journal for the Division for Early Childhood, 9* (1), 57–66.

Medway, F. J. (1989). Measuring the effectiveness of parent education. In M. J. Fine (Ed.), *The second handbook on parent education* (pp. 237–255). San Diego, CA: Academic Press.

Moran, D. R., & Whitman, T. L. (1985). The multiple effects of a play-oriented parent training program for mothers of developmentally delayed children. *Analysis and Intervention in Developmental Disabilities, 5,* 73–96.

Moreland, J. R., Schwebel, A. I., Beck, S., & Wells, R. (1982). Parents as therapists: A review of behavior therapy parent training literature—1975–1981. *Behavior Modification, 6,* 250–276.

National Center for Family-Centered Care (1990). What is family-centered care? (Brochure). Washington, DC: Association for the Care of Children's Health.

Palmer, S., & Cochran, L. (1988). Parents as agents of career development. *Journal of Counseling Psychology, 35,* 71–76.

Parks, P. L., & Smeriglio, V. L. (1986). Relationships among parenting knowledge, quality of stimulation in the home and infant development. *Family Relations, 35,* 411–416.

Rogers-Warren, A. K., & Warren, S. (1983). Facilitating early language and social development: Parents as teachers. In E. M. Goetz & A. E. Allen (Eds.), *Early childhood education: Special environmental, policy, and legal-considerations.* Rockville, MD: Aspen Systems Corp.

Schaefer, E. S. (1989). Prediction of child competence from maternal beliefs and behaviors during infancy. In C. Doxiadis (Ed.), *Early influences shaping the individual* (pp. 257–268). New York: Plenum.

Snow, C. E., & Ferguson, C. A. (Eds.) (1977). *Talking to children: Language input and acquisition.* Cambridge: Cambridge University Press.

Snow, C., Midkiff-Borunda, S., Small, A., & Proctor, A. (1984). Therapy as social interaction: Analyzing the contexts for language remediation. *Topics in Language Disorders, 4,* 72–85.

Tiegerman, E., & Siperstein, M. (1982, April). Communication training: Changing mother-child interaction. Paper presented at the meeting of the New York State Speech and Hearing Association, Ellenville, NY.

Tiegerman, E., & Siperstein, M. (1984, September). Individual patterns of interaction in the mother-child dyad: Implications for parent intervention. *Topics in Language Disorders.*

Timm, M. A., & Rule, S. (1981). RIP: A cost effective parent-implemented program for young handicapped children. *Early Development and Care, 7,* 147–163.

Turnbull, A., & Turnbull, H. R. (1982). Parent involvement in the education of handicapped children: A critique. *Mental Retardation, 20,* 115–122.

Turnbull, A. P., & Turnbull, H. R. (1986). Families, professionals and exceptionality: A special partnership. Columbus, OH: Charles E. Merrill.

Wiese, M. R. (1992). A critical review of parent training research. *Psychology in the Schools, 29,* 229–236.

Wiese, M. R., & Kramer, J. J. (1988). Parent training research: An analysis of the empirical literature 1975–1985. *Psychology in the Schools, 25,* 325–330.

Yell, M., & Espin, C. (1990). The handicapped children's protection act of 1986: Time to pay the piper? *Exceptional Children, 56,* 396–407.

CHAPTER

7

THE CLASSROOM AS LANGUAGE LABORATORY

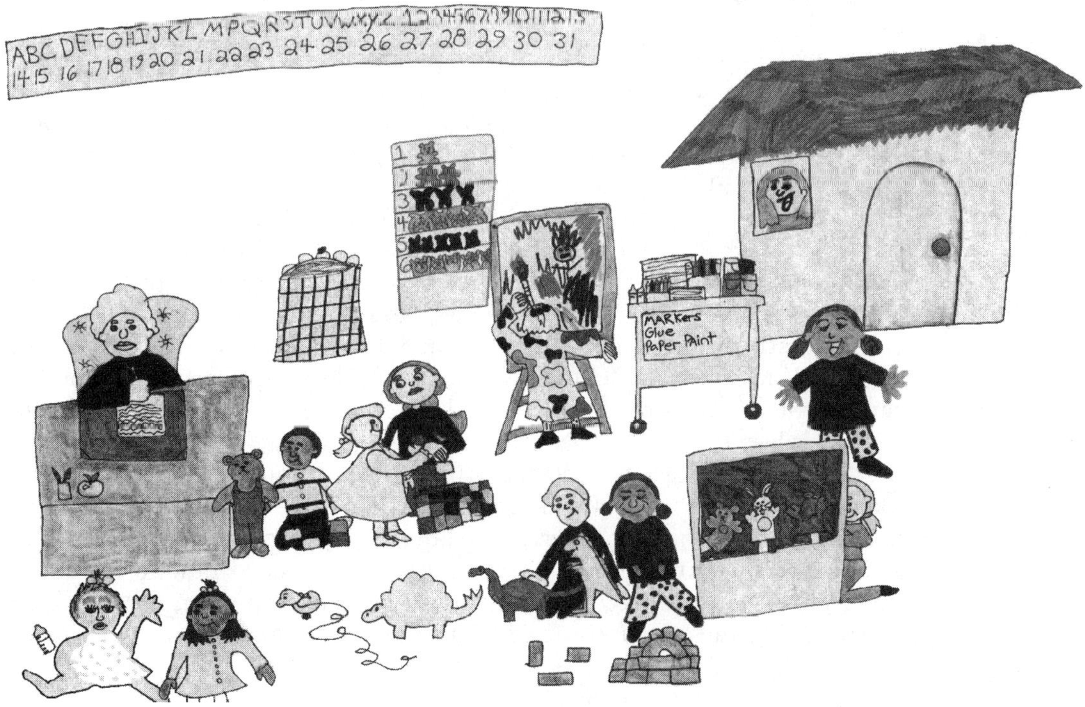

The purpose of this chapter is to highlight the relationship between pragmatic language theory and the role of the classroom in facilitating language-learning behaviors in preschool children. Children with severe language and communication disorders need to learn how to communicate in a social context. Initiating communication, staying on topic, expressing relevant ideas, describing events, and narrating a story are all representative of children in a normal nursery school environment. Children with severe language and communication disorders present production and comprehension deficits in one or more of the language component areas. Clearly, the classroom can be a context in which children can apply the concepts and structures that they have learned in individual/prescriptive therapy to a setting where other communicators can respond and provide feedback. For example, a child may develop the ability to verbally request a familiar object, such as his favorite car, in individual therapy. This skill is generalized through various social contexts in the classroom setting, when the child has an opportunity to request a car or cars in the classroom from adults and peers. If his request is not met, he must then further generalize his skills to obtain what he wants.

The classroom environment provides a variety of social and communicative interactions with both peers and adults (Hart & Rogers-Warren, 1978; Halle, Albert, & Anderson, 1984). The speech/language pathologist who functions as the primary classroom teacher creates an atmosphere that is highly structured, yet natural and spontaneous. Although activities are presented to the entire group, the teacher addresses the individual needs of each child. Thus, there is a strong collaboration between the classroom teacher and individual therapist. The speech/language pathologist who provides individual therapy addresses each child's specific needs in a direct, therapeutic manner. For example, he or she will typically plan a lesson that will trigger specific responses from the child and will concentrate on that child's goals through preconceived activities that include the adult and that child only.

In the classroom, peers and adults act as role models for social and language behaviors (Shatz, 1982). In addition, the pragmatic skills demonstrated by each child provide the foundation for the group pragmatic interactions. Because each child possesses her own strengths and weaknesses, the teacher is able to capitalize on the strengths to provide peer models for appropriate communicative behavior (McCormick & Schiefelbusch, 1990). Children learn to respond to the communicative styles of others while developing their own individual communicative style.

Learning to interact in a social setting is part of communication learning. To understand the social rules and roles that govern the interaction between communicators is an important part of the language-based educational curriculum. Preschool children with language disorders must learn how to interact with their peers. The social setting that underscores severe pragmatic problems is potentially the most important setting for learning and communication appli-

This chapter was co-authored by Rosemarie Cartusciello-King.

cation. The classroom context provides a learning to learn process. The more children with language disorders learn about the communication process, the better they function in the social setting. So the question then becomes: What are the goals and activities that facilitate interaction between children?

NATURALISTIC FACILITATION IN THE CLASSROOM

Individualizing the Classroom Setting

One of the most important issues in any classroom context is how to provide individual teaching facilitation for a language-disordered child in the context of a larger group setting. The social setting is the most important context for language learning. However, given the individual and idiosyncratic differences among children with language and communication disorders, the group setting must be offset by highly prescriptive and individualized language therapy sessions. The purpose of individual language therapy is to introduce, train, and organize specific language skills for the child. The language-group experience in the classroom provides an application and generalization experience for what he or she acquires in individual therapy. In order to become an effective language learner and user, the child must acquire a dynamic set of communicative skills while interacting, communicating, and sharing with other children in a social context. The classroom group experience provides a set of learning dynamics that individual therapy cannot provide. How does the classroom teacher individualize instruction in a group setting?

One variable that the teacher can manipulate involves different teaching strategies that can be used in a formal teaching environment. These strategies can provide a mechanism for the teacher to individualize planned daily routines to provide specific instruction for each child in the group. Classroom activities can be changed by various organizational manipulations. The teacher can individualize instruction by altering different kinds of structural aspects in the classroom:

a. the environmental structure, the organization of the actual physical setting;
b. the learning structure, the organization of activities or communicative responses expected from the child;
c. the teaching structure, the organization of the adult's language input.

Environmental Structure

In viewing the classroom environment and the degree of organizational structure in the classroom, it is important to determine whether toys, materials, and activities are so easily accessible that there is no reason for the children to use their language to request or comment. Rearranging the environment so that toys and materials are out of reach provides a factor for communicative facilitation and communicative initiation. It is also important to determine if the objects and materials in the classroom are interesting, motivating, and desirable. Objects that are attractive to children also facilitate requesting, commenting, and other communicative interactional functions. Materials must be functional and authentic so that children can make the connection between school, home, and their community.

The size of the group should also be considered in terms of environmental structure. The larger the group, the more difficult it might be for the teacher to individualize instruction for a specific child. Subgrouping and clustering children in different play settings is often very helpful. Children must learn to function communicatively and socially in various group settings and group sizes. Presenting activities first in smaller groups and then in larger ones allows the teacher to assess the child's interactional abilities as a function of the number of children.

It is often very difficult for a child who is language disordered to sit in a group of fifteen or twenty peers for half an hour paying attention, listening, and initiating appropriate communicative responses. A child's comment that is based on the teacher's interaction with another child is quite sophisticated and requires a great deal of learning in a smaller group context. The size of the environmental group must be manipulated so that the child has an opportunity to apply his language skills in successively larger and more complex settings.

Making use of naturalistic teaching opportunities presented by certain kinds of activities is also important in the environmental structure. Circle time, snack time, play time, and even toileting provide natural opportunities to facilitate language learning. These are activities that present exposure to normal social routines, not only in school but also at home, in restaurants, on playgrounds, and in other natural settings. Low-structured activities in which children are allowed to initiate and to interact based on their own decision making provide the teacher with an opportunity to act as a social-director rather than a teacher-director.

Given the communicative relationship between teacher and child, the nature of the teacher-child interaction during a highly structured lesson is quite different than that during a low-structured lesson. In a high-structured situation, the teacher often has specific goals that she has targeted for response. In a low-structured activity, she follows the child's initiations and intervenes, facilitates, and comments, rather than directing or targeting specific responses. The need for high- and low-structured activities in the classroom depends on specific language-learning goals.

The teaching strategies identified in naturally occurring adult-child interactions are often referred to as incidental teaching. In incidental teaching, the timing of these interactions is critical. In a naturally occurring interaction, behaviors are child-initiated, and the environment is arranged to create a mechanism for communication. The child's initiations represent a stimulus for the adult to respond with requests for elaborated utterances, comments, models, and imitations. The teacher provides an action in a daily routine, such as pouring milk into pudding. The child's communicative initiations can be reinforced socially by the adult's attention and responses to specific child requests.

Learning Structure

Manipulating the learning structure involves organizing activities to target specific responses and language behaviors. In teaching a child to request or ask for a specific object, the teacher may place the object out of reach, but in the child's line of vision. As the child approaches the desired object, the teacher may ask, "What do you want?" If the child does not respond or gives a minimal response, the teacher can provide a prompt or a language model for the response. The prompt level indicates how much information must be provided for the adult's model. In order to facilitate the child's response initially, the teacher may have to provide the child with the entire response—"I want the truck." As the child learns to request, the prompting becomes more minimalized so that the teacher provides less information in the model. When the child responds to the prompt, the teacher reinforces the child's approximation and gives him or her the requested object.

The use of a sequence of prompts is an important feature in all of these teaching strategies. Prompt levels may be minimalized by various fading techniques. One fading strategy is for the teacher to provide the entire model—"I want the truck." Over successive presentations of this model the teacher lowers the volume of his or her voice until it becomes a whisper. Another fading technique is to successively present less of the model. The initial prompt might be the entire sentence—"I want the truck"; in the next training sequence, "I want the . . ."; in a third sequence, even less—"I want . . . ." Eventually the entire prompt is faded out, leaving the child with the appropriate verbal response in relation to the contextual social routine.

Another learning strategy that may be used by the teacher is referred to as a time-delay strategy. This technique can best be put to use in the framework of a familiar daily routine. The child is used to performing the routine in a specific order and sequence; he learns to expect specific objects to be present and actions to occur. The time-delay strategy allows the teacher to create a natural break in the routine in order to allow the child an opportunity to initiate some communicative performance. The training begins when the child becomes aware that the routine has stopped. The teacher may be poised to pour the milk, but she waits for the child to comment. She provides a visual prompt, which is the associated action, she looks at the child, she holds out the object to the child. If the child is able to provide the appropriate language response in a reasonable period of time, he is socially reinforced by the teacher and by the continuation of the familiar routine. If the child does not respond, the teacher provides a prompt that is progressively minimalized over time. The child imitates the teacher's model, and the social routine continues.

Classroom routines are important because they provide familiarity and a framework that can be expanded, developed, and individualized. Building routines allows the child and the group a semantic framework that establishes familiar actions, semantic expressions, familiar words, and expectations as to what should come next. An important part of the classroom routine is for the teacher to do something unexpected once the routine has been established. Changing the routine, breaking the routine, or violating the routine are ways of getting children to repair the sequence and to talk about what has occurred.

Teaching Structure

As discussed earlier, just as parents utilize the principle of semantic relatedness at home, teachers are also sensitively attuned to these variables in the classroom. The teacher as a language model carefully regulates her input to the children to increase the probability for reciprocal communication. Some of the ways a teacher can regulate her own language might include modifying the length and complexity of her utterances, utilizing gestures and visual cues, and providing a hierarchy of prompt levels by modeling, physical support, and verbal elicitations (Halle, Baer, & Spradlin, 1981). Teacher-child interaction represents a communication process that must be sensitively attuned to the language comprehension skills of the child who is learning to communicate. The routine daily experiences that occur in the classroom provide a rich source for language facilitation. The teacher's input is child-sensitive, child-oriented, and contextually based.

The topic of conversation involves the daily routine or activity in the classroom (Hart & Risley, 1980). The content of the interaction is determined by the child in the classroom context or activity. By being semantically related, the teacher's input relates specifically to what the child is doing or saying during the activity; the teacher's language is directly oriented toward child performances—verbal and nonverbal. The teacher's language follows the child and, therefore, the child is in control of the topic and the content of the interaction. The teacher provides the contingency network between linguistic structure and contextual occurrences. For the child who presents with severe difficulties in mapping linguistic structures onto nonlinguistic experiences, the classroom teacher reinforces the bridge between language and the ongoing context.

The teacher also facilitates the development of specific semantic functions by utilizing expansion, extension, elicitation, imitation, and commenting techniques. In language expansion the teacher fills in grammatical aspects that have been omitted from the child's production; if, for example, the child says "Boy run," the teacher can facilitate language learning by expanding the child's utterance with "The boy is running." Here, the teacher is paying attention to the linguistic or structural aspects of the child's production. In addition, this provides the child with auditory feedback of appropriate forms in language.

In the case of extension as a semantic procedure, the teacher provides new information based on the child's language content. For example, if the child says

"The boy playing," the teacher can provide an extension based on the child's utterance with "The boy is playing in the park." This technique enhances a variety of skills, such as lexical/concept development, associations, relatedness, and semantic-syntactic forms.

By using elicitation, the teacher tries to elicit or obtain additional information from the child about the topic or activity. Here the child might say "Look, a duck," and the teacher would follow with "Tell me more about it." Another type of elicitation is questioning. The technique can be used successfully to obtain information from children who may otherwise not initiate communicative interactions or include pertinent or significant content with regard to the topic. However, caution should be taken that the child is not questioned excessively. If this occurs, he or she may feel pressured when attempting to provide responses. In addition, the environment can become less spontaneous and natural.

In an imitation activity, the goal is to tie together the linguistic utterance with a nonlinguistic performance. In this particular case, it is getting the child to "say and do" at the same time—to perform an action, and then linguistically code a performance. For example: As Michael opens his juice, the teacher provides a verbal stimulus by saying "Michael, open juice." Michael may imitate all or part of the teacher's presentation, but the goal is to reinforce him for coding verbally what he is doing. Further, the teacher can comment on observations and situations such as "Michael, your car fell." Imitation and commenting also reinforce attending skills and can highlight important aspects of the environment that a child might not otherwise notice.

The use of such semantic facilitation techniques provides the child with a rich source of related input and also underscores the reciprocal aspects of communicative interaction that must occur in conversation.

Social Routines and Contingencies

There are various activities that lend themselves to becoming social routines in the classroom; activities such as making pudding, coloring, snack time, and storytelling time provide repeated presentations from day to day. These activities are highly motivational as well as communicatively instructive in a group setting. In the framework of snack time, each child can learn to find his lunch box, sit in his chair, open his lunch box, eat and share his food items. As snack time is repeated on a daily basis, social routines—patterns of behavior—are repeated from day to day. Social routines also have social consequences. It is important for children to learn that there are consequences to behavior just as there are contingencies for learning. Children with language and communication disorders need to learn that their behaviors create reactions and responses from peers and adults. Offering a peer a cookie creates a different response than hitting a peer does.

Behavioral consequences need to be highlighted so that socially appropriate behaviors are acquired in the group setting. Children can be reinforced by means of primary reinforcers, naturally occurring events, and/or by means of verbal praise from teachers and peers. The classroom can be specifically organized to develop social routines so that violations or breaks in the routines provide opportunities for the child's communicative initiations—requests and/or comments.

The naturalistic setting provides the greatest opportunities for a form of natural learning that has the highest potential for generalization. The more familiar one setting is to another, the greater the chance that the child's language behavior will be generalized from the first to the second context. The more familiar the behavior of the adults from one setting to another, the greater the opportunity for the child's language behavior to generalize from one person to another. Generalization is a critical application to classroom instruction. Behaviors that are learned in individual therapy and in school may not generalize to the outside world or to the home. The classroom teacher needs to utilize naturalistic techniques and learning routines to ensure that language behaviors will generalize across the curriculum and across settings.

Classroom Themes

Because the classroom is organized with objects, people, and activities that relate to the functioning abilities of the children, the level of complexity of the classroom is related to the group's level of comprehension (Hart & Risley, 1974, 1975, 1986). As the group becomes more sophisticated, the classroom activities and facilitated language skills become more complex. The general knowledge learning is accomplished by means of activities that teach children how to use objects and how to interact while objects are being used. An emphasis is placed on teaching children to talk about their actions during an activity. In addition, children are reinforced by helping a peer, initiating an interaction with a peer, and maintaining an interaction with a peer. Activities are repeated over the course of several weeks so that the routines become familiar. Each week there is a theme—a holiday, the season, someone's birthday—around which daily activities are related. The theme provides a mechanism for relating information, knowledge, objects, and actions and allows the teacher to develop vocabulary and semantic functions.

Themes provide a meaningful bridge between addressing each child's specific language goals and presenting group lessons that provide numerous opportunities for each child to achieve his or her goals. Themes become even more meaningful when they are initiated by the children. Child-directed themes can improve motivational levels and interest levels; children may be more eager to participate in activities as the content becomes more functional and related to their lives. Activity sheets are sent home on a daily basis so that parents can duplicate experiences at home and talk to children about activities that occurred during the day.

Facilitating Interaction

At the beginning of the school year or when organizing a class for the first time, the first issue to be considered should be the size of the class. Obviously, the number of students affects the quantity and the quality of interactions among the children and between the teacher and each child. Although classes may vary from six to fifteen students, it is more productive to keep the class size small. The smaller the class, the greater the opportunity will be for interactions to occur among peers and for each child to receive individual attention. A small class allows each child to familiarize himself with his peers and with his teachers. Communicative interactions can be closely monitored and regulated by the teacher—interactions between teacher and child, teacher and children, child and child, child and children, and children and children.

Child-Child Interaction

The child-child interaction that is critical to social development can be facilitated in the classroom when the teacher, acting as a director, reinforces one child for playing with or talking to another. The teacher can reinforce these interactions through such responses as direct verbal praise ("Good, you asked for the car"); approving the interaction ("I like the way you waited for your turn"); acknowledging that the communicative intent was achieved; and pointing out the appropriate interaction to the other children in the group. The basic approach in the classroom is clearly pragmatic.

Classroom activities are organized to facilitate interaction between children: having one child give another child a toy, having each child take a turn in a cooking activity, setting up daily routines and giving each child a part of the routine to follow and complete. Each routine can consist of a communication script that is used on a daily basis. These scripts include the sequence of events for each routine, expected verbal and social interactions, appropriate pragmatic behaviors, and specific content areas that need to be addressed (e.g., vocabulary, following directions, etc.). Children become familiar with these scripts and routines as they begin to participate in them independently. If they do not change the script, the teacher can do so by extending or altering the expected routine to facilitate language development.

The teacher can facilitate language between children in many different ways by using procedures such as modeling, imitation, and generalization learning. In modeling an interaction, the teacher might tell Michael what to say to Stephen and then reinforce each child for the communication interaction that occurs. In time, the outcome of the interactions begins to function as reinforcement (McLean & Vincent, 1984). The teacher always starts at the child's level of communication functioning, even if that level is a gesture. In successive activities, the teacher can increase the complexity of the linguistic model so that she is always providing a language representation that is more complex than the child's. As a speech/language pathologist, the teacher can pinpoint the level at which the child has mastered a particular language skill. She will then provide a delicate balance between what has been mastered and the next-level language skill to be achieved. Success is experienced at a higher level; the child is not set up for failure.

Generalization

Watson and Lord (1982) indicate that there is a difference between the knowledge acquired in a one-to-one therapeutic context and the ability to use that knowledge appropriately in everyday situations. Because the classroom is a primary learning context, it is important for the classroom teacher to know what each child is learning in individual therapy. Vocabulary, pragmatic functions, syntactic structures, and phonological skills can all be generalized in the classroom, which provides a context in which children can exercise and practice what they know with their peers. The response and reactions of those peers can teach them to regulate, modify, and change their own language productions.

Understanding how language is used and how to facilitate language usage in the classroom is just as important as acquiring the language knowledge (Rogers-Warren & Warren, 1980; Warren & Kaiser, 1988). Teaching linguistic form is only part of the language process. The classroom provides a forum for developing the child's awareness of herself as a social communicator, in terms of her responsibility in the communication exchange. Two primary objectives should be met in the classroom: first, to expand on the communication skills that the child has in her language repertoire; and second, to generalize the child's language abilities from individual therapy (adult-child dyad) to the classroom (child-child dyad). This second objective involves teaching the child to use the social setting as a means for further learning. It is difficult for an adult to simulate being a child in a class of three-year-olds, but by facilitating and directing dyadic interactions between peers, the teacher can stimulate the social learning process step by step. The social tapestry, a complex mosaic of behaviors and skills, can be constructed in the classroom for the language-disordered child. Each child potentially can function as a speaker-initiator and a speaker-responder. The individual therapy setting cannot possibly take the place of a group of twelve child communicators.

CREATING A CHANGE IN THE CLASSROOM

A laboratory is a place for experimentation and research. Experimentation is an action or process that is undertaken to discover something not yet known or to examine something that is known and find whether or not it is effective. Each child in the language laboratory possesses a unique learning style that must be identified by the teacher so that strategies may be established and implemented to facilitate the acquisition of delayed language skills. These strategies accommodate the individual needs and style of each child. Research is the careful, patient, systematic, diligent inquiry or examination to collect facts about a particular subject. In the language laboratory, *research* refers to the on-going assessment that helps the teacher determine which development skills each child has and does not have. The classroom that reflects a language laboratory must be designed to facilitate each child's language development and all other areas of development in a naturalistic, spontaneous, motivating, social, and supportive environment. Furthermore, a structured environment consisting of routines and daily lessons that are related and meaningful for children is necessary for language learning.

A Typical Day in a Half-Day Preschool Program

Time	Activity
8:30	Children Arrive Play Time
9:00	"Hello" Song Jobs/Weather/Calendar Sharing Time
9:20	Gross-Motor Activities Aerobics for Kids Pop Goes the Weasel Stretching Exercises
9:30	Thematic Language Lesson
10:00	Special Art, Gym, or Movement Music, Auditory Training
10:30	Snack
10:50	Story Time
11:00	Thematic Language Lesson
11:30	Goodbye/Review/Prepare for Home

Goals

During each activity, a wide variety of goals are addressed and individualized according to the needs of each child. For example, if one of the primary goals is to follow directions, the teacher might individualize the directions for each child. She might use simple, one-step routine directions with John, while Mary might be presented with two-step directions that include newly acquired concepts. In addition to the individualization of goals, each child requires different prompts in order to achieve his goals. For example, John may need physical or gestural prompts to respond appropriately to the direction "Throw it away," while Mary may only need visual prompts to respond appropriately to the direction "Push the car under the bridge."

There are a variety of prompts that can be provided to elicit appropriate responses and verbalizations. These prompts are utilized by teachers in order to help children experience success and achieve their goals. (See Figure 7-1 for a list of commonly used prompts.) These prompts may be used in isolation or in combinations. When teachers utilize prompts, it is interesting to note that children become familiar with prompting and utilize these prompts with each other.

Since each child presents with his or her own language profile and own goals, it can be beneficial for the teacher to design a format that will chart goals for the group. Such a format is provided in Figure 7-2. In addition, the speech/language pathologist who provides group services may find this format helpful.

Figure 7-1
Prompts to Elicit Responses

Prompt	Example
1. Physical Prompts	Hand–over–hand Touch–Cue
2. Verbal Prompts	
Modeling	Performing an action and verbalization for imitation: Tell John, "It's my turn."
Questioning	"What do you need?"
Cloze Questioning	"The dog has a _____."
Clarification/Modification	Revising/Regulating verbal input: "Give the ball to her." "Give the ball to Mary."
Associations	"It goes with a toothbrush."
Descriptions	"It's an animal with wings that can fly."
Negations	"It's not hot, it's _____."
Repetitions	Repeating verbal input: I said, "Put the crayons in the box."
3. Phonemic Prompts	"You sleep in a b_____."
4. Gestures	Pointing Facial expressions Iconic movements: (Hand movements: big=hands wide apart) Pantomime: performing an action
5. Choices	Presentation of two choices . . . three choices . . . four choices . . . etc.
6. Visual Prompts	Objects Pictures Photographs

Figure 7-2
Sample Group Goals

Name of Child		Pragmatic						Semantic						Morpho-Syntactic				Phonological			
		E.G.	C.T.T.	P.P.	P.F.	T.M.		F.D.	V.D.	A.Q.	S.S.	N.S.		MLU	P.P.	Pr. I		FCD	B	F	WSD
John																					
Chris																					
Bobby																					
Jackie																					
Mary																					
Jill																					
Sam																					
Pavan																					
Roberto																					
Thomas																					

E.G. Eye gaze
C.T.T. Conversational turntaking
P.P. Physical proximity
P.F. Pragmatic functions
T.M. Topic maintenance

F.D. Following directions
V.D. Vocabulary development
A.Q. Answering questions
S.S. Sequencing skills
N.S. Narrative skills

MLU MLU
P.P. Present progressive
Pr. I Pronoun I

FCD Final /Con. deletion
B Backing
F Fronting
WSD Weak syllable deletion

● Skill Area — A check in the skill area represents that this is a goal for the child.

○ Prompt Level — Abbreviations of prompt levels should be used. Brief notes can be included in the spaces provided.

Categories of skill areas should include the sum of all goals for each child and should not be limited to language areas. This chart can be used for the child's present level of performance or for the documentation of results following the end of a lesson, day, or week.

Each child's goals are addressed throughout the day in each classroom activity. In the individual setting, the child's IEP goals are addressed and specific goals may be selected for each activity. The speech/language pathologist creates situations that elicit targeted skills. Even though specific goals may be emphasized in a therapy session, the SLP consistently takes every opportunity to facilitate all areas of impaired language skills, and generates documentation of trial and error, success and/or failure. A format for documenting results might include specific goals and objectives, activities, and results. It is understood that the teacher and the individual SLP must monitor, amend, and task-analyze the goals on each IEP as needed. Task analysis refers to the breakdown of a goal into its smaller component parts.

Collaboration between the classroom teacher, the individual SLP, and any team member is critical to the successful generalization of skills. Parents must be informed of their child's learning style, language profile, and the teacher's use of prompts and methods; it is also helpful if weekly activity sheets regarding themes, activities, and goals are provided. Parents must receive training to facilitate language at home by utilizing familiar daily routines or special events that occur in a natural spontaneous way in the home.

Since the routines at home are most familiar to children, parents often report progress regarding specific skills that are demonstrated in the home. It is not uncommon that these skills may not be simultaneously observed by the teaching team in school. Furthermore, it is often observed that specific skills are achieved in individual speech before they are demonstrated in the classroom setting. This is not always the case, since children may feel more familiar or comfortable in the classroom and excel there first.

The relationship between the teacher, the SLP, other team members, and the parents must be established in order to share knowledge and information regarding the child. Figure 7-3 depicts the integration of parents, the individual SLP, and the classroom teacher for the facilitating and generalization of language skills in a classroom-language laboratory. Figure 7-4 depicts a multidisciplinary approach to collaboration that places the child in the nucleus, surrounded by those who have an impact on the facilitation and generalization of goals.

An important part of collaborative efforts is sharing themes and exposing children to various contexts and situations so that they have an opportunity to generalize their skills across disciplines. Thematic units provide a common ground for all team members and can certainly be utilized by individual SLPs. Themes should be meaningful, functional, relevant, and motivating for children. In the classroom laboratory, the teacher and the children select a theme or topic of interest, which will be the focus of language activities in the classroom and in individual speech. For example, if the theme in the classroom is "All About Me," the teacher might focus on identifying special traits regarding each child and the similarities and differences among the children. The individual SLP shares the theme, but concentrates on specific goals and

Figure 7-3
Collaboration in a Classroom-Language Laboratory. Each group interfaces with the other and all have an impact on the facilitation and generalization of the child's language skills (shaded area).

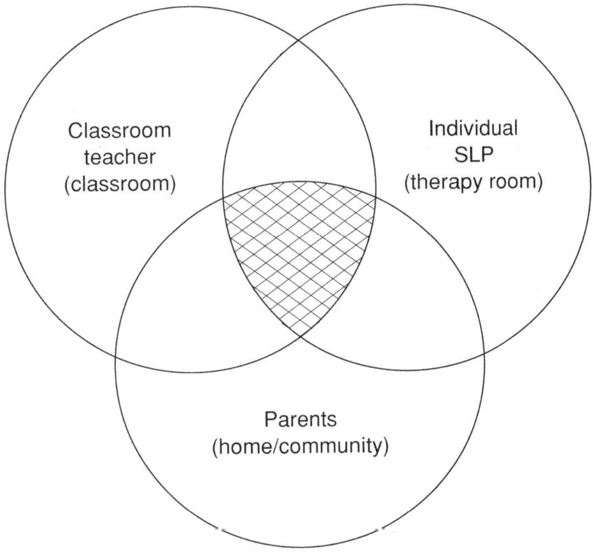

skills that are necessary for the child to be fully engaged in the group experience. Goals that would be addressed within an MLU of 3.5 might include concept development of same and different, encoding attributes (hair color, height), identifying body parts, and/or producing the final sounds in words related to the theme.

Figure 7-4
Collaboration in a Multidisciplinary Approach. Each group works closely with the child so that a holistic model for learning is achieved. Child is the core and all team members, who represent a variety of developmental areas, are consistent in the goals and procedures they implement.

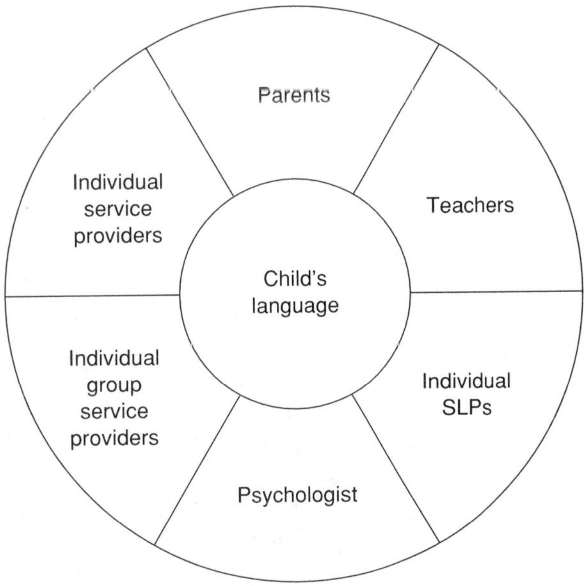

Common Themes Used in Preschool Language Programs

1. Going to School
2. All About Me
3. Fire Prevention Week
4. Seasonal and Holiday Themes
5. Community Helpers
6. Shopping for Clothes, Toys, Food, etc.
7. Eating in a Restaurant
8. Pets
9. Plants
10. Seashore

There are similarities and differences between the classroom language laboratory and the individual speech session. Both environments focus on facilitating language at the level of each child. Due to the group dynamics in the classroom, children are exposed to a variety of spontaneous creative contexts that may be initiated and responded to by adults and peers alike. The individual setting addresses specific goals and provides an extended period of time in which the child alone is engaged in a direct interaction. Although the SLP targets skills and sets up scenarios to elicit specific language, the individual setting should also be considered child-centered with adult regulation. It is quite common that children who demonstrate management difficulties in the classroom do not demonstrate these behaviors to the same extent during individual speech.

Push-In Model

Traditionally, the individual SLP pulls children out of the classroom to provide services; with a push-in model, the SLP comes into the classroom. The quality of this service may be different in each program. The SLP may conduct a group lesson and co-teach with the classroom teacher. The two professionals can interact with each other to model the behavior and language skills they are targeting. In some cases, the SLP will provide individual attention to the child during a group lesson; she will sit with the child and guide him through the group lesson while facilitating language skills. Individual services can also be provided in the corner of a classroom. Caution must be used when push-in is utilized, since this may not be a replacement for the dyadic interaction that occurs between the SLP and the child in individual therapy.

INCLUSION

With the passage of PL 94-142 in 1975, many education agencies have responded to the LRE (Least Restrictive Environment) mandate by attempting to provide physical integration for children with disabilities in public schools (Deshler, Alley, & Carlson, 1980). Inclusion, meaning the integration of disabled and nondisabled children in the educational system, is particularly important during early intervention and in early childhood special education. The legal rationale underlying the practice of inclusion, or mainstreaming, has been underscored by the passage of the Individuals with Disabilities Education Act (IDEA, Part 4) civil rights legislation, and the Americans with Disabilities Act (ADA). These laws support the rights of young children with developmental disabilities to participate in normalized educational environments such as nursery schools, preschools, and day-care centers along with children who are not disabled.

Many parents and professionals support the significance of providing the earliest possible intervention to preschool children with disabilities in settings that also serve nondisabled children. Both parents and professionals point out the difficulty of beginning this process in later school years when the developmental difficulties among children are much more difficult to address and to bridge. The emphasis, therefore, in the legislation is to begin the process of inclusion during the preschool years when parents and professionals can work together toward their educational goal (Odom & McEvoy, 1988).

Inclusion Models

There are many ways of achieving inclusion for preschool children with disabilities (McEvoy, Shores, Wehby, Johnson, & Fox, 1990). One option is to provide specialized services or itinerant services in community-based nursery schools or Head Start programs. This option places the disabled child in a regular or normalized environment from the start, allowing immediate immersion into a normalized play context. Although the language-disordered child receives only related and minimal itinerant services outside the classroom without the benefit of a special education curriculum and teacher in the classroom, it might provide an option for a mildly disabled child who does not require intensive special education services.

Another option is provided by center-based special education programs, which allow for a range of programming and services from most to least restrictive: small intensive groupings that become progressively larger as the child becomes a more sophisticated communicator. The theoretical premise here is that the least restrictive environment is the placement that meets the individual needs of the child; it would not necessarily be a regular classroom if the child were not ready for it. Along this continuum of services and programs the last step would be an inclusion or integrated classroom that would provide the disabled child with an opportunity for normalized interaction with nondisabled peers. The benefit here is that the child with the disability would begin the educational process in a self-contained intensive special education classroom, then would move along the mainstream continuum as rapidly as he or she progressed.

Clearly, there are advantages and disadvantages to each of these educational approaches; neither meets the needs of all children with language disorders. Each makes a contribution to a segment of the disabled population depending on the child's individual learning abilities. Special education has come a long way since 1975 when the original legislation, Public Law 94-142, was passed. Over the past two decades the emphasis in special education has been on specialization—providing as many different services as possible. Along with specialization came individualized programming, special education instructors, highly specialized curricula, and self-contained programming; the primary goal was to meet the individual needs of each and every disabled child. With the introduction of mainstreaming and Least Restrictive Environment in the federal legislation in 1986, the pendulum began to swing in the other direction (Peck, Richarz, Peterson, Hayden, Mineur, & Wandschneider, 1989). The Least Restrictive Environment was no longer the place that met the individual needs of the child; it was instead the regular education classroom.

Redefining LRE

In redefining Least Restrictive Environment for the disabled child, the emphasis is now on placing *all* children with disabilities in integrated, or inclusion, classrooms. As education changes and shifts its focus to the regular classroom, it is important not to lose sight of the contributions made by special education over the past two decades (Hamblin-Wilson & Thurman, 1990). The regular or normalized setting may not be possible for all disabled children, although the emphasis is to move in that direction. It would be devastating for the children and their families to be placed in a regular environment and then fail.

It becomes critical to appropriately evaluate and assess which path to take in the preschool years. To place every language-disordered preschool child in a mainstream setting denies the individual learning needs and individual learning styles of developmentally disabled children. This is not a single population; there are many different categorical groups of language-disordered children with many different needs. In addition, it is important to monitor child outcomes as education moves forward to inclusion. The educational system needs to develop criteria that will alert professionals to the fact that a child is having difficulty in an integrated classroom and requires programming as an alternative to regular education.

If inclusion programs are to exist in regular education, regular classroom teachers must be given intensive training in order to create effective classrooms in which all students will achieve their own success. Furthermore, if classrooms reflect a traditional philosophy of education, the structure of these classrooms must be altered and curricula must be adapted to accommodate the needs of all children. In the educational system today, preschool programs and early grade schools tend to educate the whole child. This includes focusing on a variety of developmental areas, such as cognitive functioning, speech and language development, gross- and fine-motor development, and social-emotional growth.

Professionals from different disciplines often work closely together, utilizing an interdisciplinary or transdisciplinary approach to educating the young child. As the child becomes older and transitions into middle school and high school, education becomes departmentalized and there is less or no collaboration between professionals working with the same child/student. Clearly, there are two separate approaches for preschool, primary, and secondary education. Since preschool programs and primary grade levels use a strong collaborative model and consist of environments that promote learning in all areas, inclusion programs would most likely experience quicker success with the younger population.

Family Factor

Just as each child is unique, each family is also unique. As we begin to utilize an ecological approach to the classroom and to the family, education must take the time to evaluate the needs of a growing multicultural population. The family, as we have discussed earlier, needs to take an active part in the educational process and learning for the child. The family's abilities, struggles, concerns, and weaknesses must be taken into consideration and their ability to understand the child's needs and provide a stimulating learning environment must be assessed by educators. As working members of the educational team, families are subjected to emotional, social, economic, and psychological difficulties. The child as a member of the family will be affected by the family's outlook, commitment, and emotional health. The classroom is not just for the child. The classroom is for the family and to be shared by all who work with the child. The truly natural setting is the home because it represents the child's primary setting. In developing inclusion, educators must take into consideration the struggles of the family. Inclusion will only be successful if the family is mobilized to contribute. The family is the critical force in the life of the child and needs to be assessed in terms of its cultural beliefs, family structure, and emotional struggles.

FACILITATING SOCIALIZATION

McEvoy and colleagues (1990) suggest that the physical proximity of disabled and nondisabled children in relation to one another will not ensure that both populations will actually interact. Specifically, providing a physical context only provides the possibility that they will accidentally share the same space, but does not ensure that these two populations have the skills to successfully socialize with each other. These researchers suggest that successful social integration can only occur with direct intervention from teachers and administrators and parents. In addition, it is not clear what methodological procedures can be used to successfully achieve socialization in various communities, in various cultural settings, and with various disabled populations. They suggest that several variables must be considered in order to begin the socialization process between disabled and nondisabled children. These include (a) peer training, (b) organization of the classroom, and (c) attitudinal contingencies.

Perhaps one of the most important issues presented by these researchers is that the classroom represents an ecological environment that facilitates the social learning process between disabled and nondisabled children. The variables that contribute to the ecology must be understood and appropriately factored in. To assume that the mere placement of disabled children in a regular classroom will successfully achieve mainstreaming or integration is rather naive.

Peer Partners

Underlying the theoretical premise of peer facilitation is that children can learn from one another (Fenrick, Pearson, & Pepelnjak, 1984; Guaralnick, 1986). In the process of mainstreaming children with disabilities into a normalized classroom environment, educators have considered how normal children can serve as models for the disabled (Raab, Nordquist, Cunningham, & Bleim, 1986). In this case we are considering the preschool population, indicating that even at ages three and four disabled and nondisabled children can socialize and play together.

By the age of three, the normal child has a wealth of social, communicative language and cognitive skills. By the age of four, pragmatic, semantic, and syntactic skills are not only emerging in the normal child but are well on the way toward integration of the entire linguistic system. The normal child can function as a language facilitator and peer socializer. The disordered child, particularly the language-disordered child, presents with one or more deficits in the language component areas. The normal preschooler can serve as a model by filling in many of the developmental gaps for the language-disordered child, for whom the best learning experience involves the opportunity for language learning and language practice in a social setting (Odom, Hoyson, Jamieson, & Strain, 1985). Clearly, nothing can take the place of a social experience that consists of other children playing, interacting, talking, and exploring. The issue becomes the structure of the environment itself.

Typically speaking, nondisabled children would not necessarily include a learner with a disability. Children clearly socialize along a hierarchy that involves a set of competencies and skills. The most socially competent children play together and function in a group together; children who are less socially competent are excluded and usually form their own group. Social skills are primarily acquired through learning, observation, modeling, and practice. Children learn very early in the first twenty-four months of life that there are specific behaviors that elicit social responsiveness from others. Social skills are not developed in a vacuum; they must be developed in steps of increasing difficulty.

Learning to interact and communicate in a social dyad is a first step in the socialization process. Eventually, however, children must learn to function communicatively in a larger group context. They must learn to be aware of play themes, peers, roles, and rules that govern a group dynamic experience. For the child with language disorders, this presents a monumental problem. Deficits in pragmatic, semantic, and syntactic areas limit the language-disordered child's ability to learn the rules of play, to initiate interactions, to maintain conversations, to describe events, and to share stories. The child who is less communicatively competent will be less socially competent and, therefore, will have much less of an opportunity to function with normal peers on the playground.

The classroom provides a mechanism for a systematic progression of social experiences (Guaralnick, 1986). For the language-disordered child the progression can begin with a single peer or friend and ultimately progress to integration and socialization in the larger group. McEvoy and colleagues (1990) indicate that nondisabled children must be formally trained as peer facilitators for children with disabilities. Clearly, the language-disordered child does not have the social interactional abilities to initiate a conversation, an activity, or an interaction. The initiation must therefore come from the nondisabled child. In the case of preschool children, there are several techniques that the teacher can use to develop interaction between disabled and nondisabled children.

The teacher might develop a buddy system in which a child with a language disorder and a normal child are assigned to one another. The normal child should be encouraged to initiate play activities with his or her partner. The teacher should reinforce all approaching, offering, sharing, and maintaining play behaviors by the normal child. The nondisabled peer can be told, "Here, take this toy over to Michael and give it to him." When she accomplishes the selected behavior, she should be verbally reinforced by the teacher. Interactional initiations produced by the nondisabled child in relation to her partner can be selectively reinforced. As she produces an increasing number of interactional behaviors oriented toward her partner, behavioral and social changes in the child with the disability can also be measured and analyzed.

In functioning as a director, the teacher can modify the normal child's social behaviors so that they more effectively influence the language-disordered child's social responses. Once this goal has been accomplished, maintenance of the interaction (i.e., increasing the number of turns or exchanges) between the two children over a sustained period of time can become the goal. This working dyad between peers places the nondisabled child in a leadership position that uniquely sensitizes her to the needs of her partner. The dyad serves the learning needs of the disabled child by providing a means for socialization instruction that is highly specialized.

The Classroom Environment

The organization of the classroom must facilitate the learning process as children—disabled and nondisabled—learn to interact socially. The classroom must offer toys and activities that promote social interaction. Beckman and Kohl (1984) describe the kinds of objects and toys that can be used in a classroom as either socially facilitating or isolating. Corners of the classroom can be organized with specific themes in mind. Large objects and manipulanda provide a continual source of novelty and play. As the nondisabled children become interested in toys and activities, they will encourage their disabled partners. At this stage, the teacher can provide direct prompts and praise for the interaction occurring between children, and can also encourage children to move from one play corner to another, keeping the movement and activity as a primary means for facilitating social interaction.

ATTITUDES

Peck, Hayden, Wandschneider, Peterson, and Richarz (1989) describe the specific concerns expressed by parents, teachers, and administrators regarding integrated programming (see Figure 7-5).

Parents' Concerns

The concerns of parents of children with disabilities include

- the preparation and ability of teachers to accomplish mainstreaming in the classroom (Reichart, Lynch, Anderson, Svobodny, DiCola, & Mercury, 1989)
- whether early childhood teachers have specific training in special education. Does the early childhood teacher understand developmental disabilities, and how to remediate those disabilities in a regular classroom?
- the possibility that early childhood teachers cannot manage behavioral problems and that there are too many children in the regular preschool program
- the possibility that the nondisabled children will ridicule or exclude the children with disabilities
- the preconceived attitudes that the parents of nondisabled children may have, and how those attitudes will impact on all children (Schaefer, 1989; Sparling & Lowman, 1983)

Figure 7-5
Concerns and Fears

Parents of Children with Disabilities

1. I am afraid that my child will be rejected by the nondisabled children in the classroom.
2. I am afraid that my child will be picked on by the nondisabled children in the classroom.
3. I am afraid that the teacher does not know anything about developmental disabilities.
4. I am afraid that my disabled child will not get enough individual attention.
5. I am afraid that the philosophy of inclusion is really a smokescreen for schools' not providing individual therapeutic services for children with disabilities.

Parents of Nondisabled Children

1. I am afraid that children with disabilities in the classroom will negatively affect my child's learning.
2. I am afraid that the teacher will spend too much time paying attention to the children with disabilities in the classroom.
3. There are too many children with disabilities in the classroom.
4. I am afraid that the learning of the entire class is going to be slowed down by the children with disabilities in the classroom.
5. I am afraid that there are too many levels of learning ability in the room, and the teacher will not be able to address the needs of each child.

Parents of nondisabled children also have concerns (Green & Stoneman, 1989)

- How will their children be affected by the developmentally disabled children in the room?
- Will teachers pay too much attention to the disabled children? Will their children will be neglected, ignored, and receive much less attention?

Both sets of parents are concerned about the possibility that as the class gets significantly larger, the individual needs of the children will be ignored.

Figure 7-5 describes parents' fears about the inclusion process. It is clear that unless these fears are addressed, the inclusion process will not be easily or readily accomplished.

Teachers' Concerns

Early childhood teachers' concerns include

- the fact that they have not received sufficient training to understand or to meet the needs of developmentally disabled children
- the fact that they do not know *how* to accomplish mainstreaming and integration in the classroom, specifically how to teach disabled and

nondisabled children to socialize, interact, and communicate with each other

- the possibility that there are too many language-disordered children in the classroom. How many children with disabilities can be introduced into a regular classroom without disrupting the educational process?
- having enough support from administrators, related staff, and parents
- the need for ongoing instructional development outside of the classroom

Clearly, there is a need for staff development; inclusion programming is so new and the methodological procedures to achieve it are unfamiliar. Staff development must be incorporated into the curriculum of any program. All members of the staff should be part of the training efforts to achieve the inclusion philosophy and to meet the needs of individual children. Regular education teachers should receive intensive training on developmental disabilities. This is critical, since early childhood teachers often feel overwhelmed by having developmentally disabled children in their classrooms. If inclusion remains a staff effort, the collaboration of professionals provides support for each individual member. Inclusion can be effective only if parents and teachers are committed to its success. Collaboration allows for ongoing monitoring and modification; it is this communication between the significant parties that will allow for the educational adjustments that will benefit all of the children.

Administrators

Administrators are concerned about accomplishing the goals related to inclusion. They see that inclusion is a final step, but there are many important programmatic aspects that must be resolved to ensure the success of the inclusion philosophy. The teachers must be trained, the parents must be educated, and the nondisabled children must be readied before language-disordered children are introduced into the regular classroom. Administrators are also concerned about the development of a preschool curriculum that takes into account the inclusion process. Finally, they are most sensitive to the attitudes and concerns of their teachers and staff. If teachers are opposed to the introduction of disabled children into their classrooms, the administrators must work to change these attitudes or the inclusion process will not be successful.

Classroom Clusters

As we have discussed above, the classroom represents the primary domain for language learning. How should children be clustered? One way is to assign children to classrooms by age. However, since there may be a marked discrepancy between a child's chronological age and his mental age or level of functioning, this is not the most efficacious criterion for classroom assignment. Another approach to assigning children to classrooms is by category or disabling condition. Children diagnosed as mentally retarded go into one classroom; children diagnosed as language disordered or deaf go into separate classrooms. Categorical placement such as this also presents problems, since children with the same disabling condition can present with very different learning styles and be at very different developmental levels.

Another possibility is to group children based on their language abilities. Children with similar language problems can be placed in the same classroom. One way to do this is to develop a language profile for each classroom (see Figure 7-6). For example, children with pragmatic deficits might go into one

Figure 7-6
Language Component Analysis: Child Profile

Child's Name:____________________
Child's Chronological Age:____________

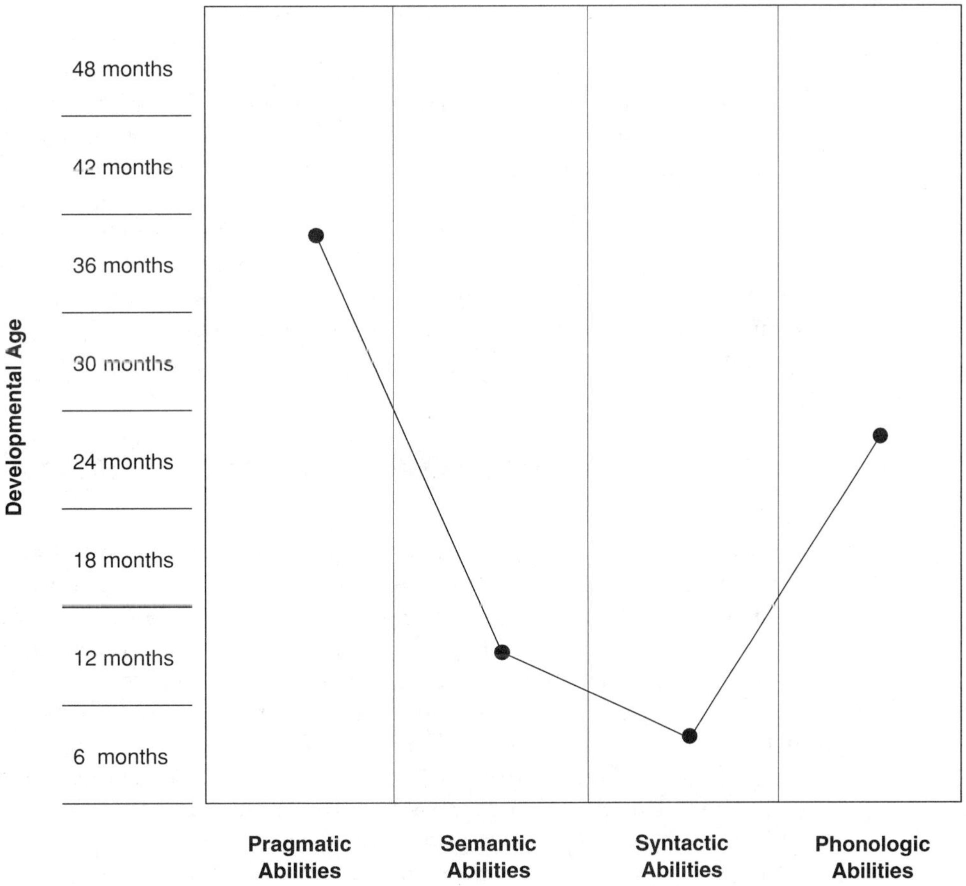

classroom and children with semantic problems into another. Each classroom represents a different language component area, and the children assigned to that classroom present with primary deficits in that language component area. This would also provide the teacher with a focus for educational and linguistic instruction. If the children present with pragmatic deficits, then language learning in the classroom focuses on the development of pragmatic communicative skills in children.

Another issue related to clusters involves subgrouping children in the room with a teacher and two teaching assistants. A group of twelve or fifteen children can be subgrouped for specific activities into groups of four or five, allowing for more direct adult-child input and interaction. This also provides for a much greater opportunity for each child to verbalize and/or communicate with members of his or her peer group and the adult or teacher. The school year could begin with children functioning in smaller subgroups; as the year progresses, activities could include two or more of these clusters consisting of ten or fifteen children together. By the end of the year, the entire class could participate as a group. Finally, children can be clustered in a group of twelve or fifteen through seating arrangements that place them according to their strengths and weaknesses. In addition, teachers and teacher assistants position themselves according to each child's specific needs (see Figure 7-7).

The classroom in which a speech/language pathologist is the primary classroom teacher is similar to if not the same as a classroom utilizing the whole-language philosophy. Materials and play areas may be the same as those found in traditional classrooms; however, the way in which the materials and sections are utilized to facilitate language is clearly different. The classroom functions as a language laboratory and can be described as the place where the language skills of each child are analyzed and each child is challenged to progress at his or her own pace. It is a finely tuned environment that emphasizes the realization of each child's communicative potential.

THE ECOLOGY OF COMMUNICATION

In the last several chapters and in this chapter, a multitude of problems have been discussed. An important issue facing education today is mainstreaming. The attitudes, concerns, and worries about mainstreaming must be addressed by means of a working model in school systems—a communication model that can be utilized effectively for parents, teachers, and children. Clearly, if these attitudes and concerns are not addressed, mainstreaming will never be effectively achieved. Parents of nondisabled children cannot be forced to place their preschool children into a "mixed classroom." They must be helped to understand that the mainstreaming process benefits their children as well as the disabled children—in the classroom and on the playground.

Regular education teachers must overcome their fears of the disabled and

Figure 7-7
In the Classroom-Language Laboratory, Teacher and Teacher Assistant Positioning According to Each Child's Needs.

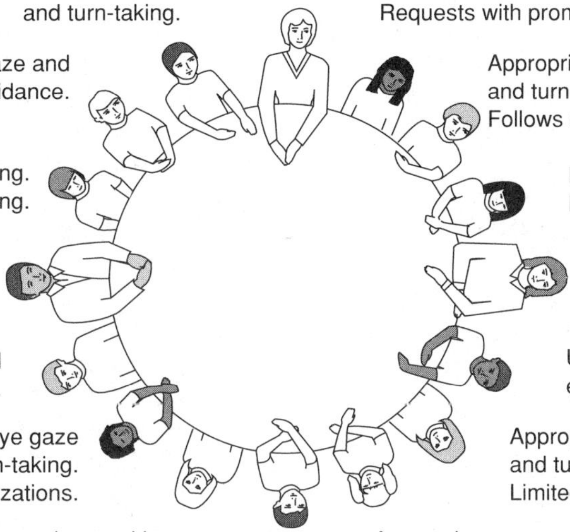

must receive additional academic training as well as ongoing staff development. Administrators must learn how to facilitate the personal growth in teachers and the open communication between parents and teachers. There should be an ongoing discussion group or forum in which parents and teachers can express their concerns and attitudes about the direction of this new curriculum. How should parents and teachers be taught? Where and when should this discussion group meet? How should problems that arise with and between parents of nondisabled children and regular education teachers be addressed on an ongoing basis so that all benefit?

It is clearly important to look at the mainstream process from a holistic prospective—as an ecological environment that requires the input of all of the variables contributing to one single goal. If mainstreaming is going to succeed, then all of the individuals should contribute to the process; parents of language-disordered children, parents of normal children, teachers, disabled children, and nondisabled children must all understand the common goal, the learning process, and the benefits. All of us are invested in the success of inclusion. All of us must know that each of us has something to learn; each of us must be part of the decision-making process.

SUMMARY

This chapter described how the classroom provides the most important aspect for language learning for preschool children with language disorders. As an instructional setting, the classroom allows the child, the teacher, and the parent to come together with a common goal—language learning. Ultimately, the classroom represents the transitional setting for the child to function in the mainstream environment. For many preschool language-disordered children, the inclusion classroom is not the appropriate initial setting; the overwhelming learning aspects and complexities of the integrated context emphasize many problems. It is important, therefore, to understand the language-disordered child's language-learning level in order to educate him along a continuum of more inclusive socialization experiences.

The classroom as a language laboratory includes many different learning variables that must be incorporated into educational instruction. The classroom teacher must be aware of the child and the facilitation procedures that will accommodate language learning. The classroom provides a mechanism for individual, dyadic, small-group, and large-group learning experiences, all of which will be necessary for the language-disordered child to function in the integrated classroom, the regular classroom, and the real world.

A FEW WORDS FROM TOYA DAVIS

This chapter was about the function of the classroom in developing skills in language-disordered children. I never missed an opportunity to watch Jonathan on the closed-circuit video system. I have always felt that parents should have an opportunity to watch the interaction between the teacher and the children. The classroom is truly a laboratory for learning. In watching Jonathan on a weekly basis, I saw my son in a very different situation than the one provided at home. I saw him with peers in many situations, during many different activities. At times I was struck by the fact that I saw many sides of Jonathan that I did not see at home. In observing the classroom I learned not only about Jonathan as a learner but also about the techniques that were successful in teaching him. After observing Jonathan in class I could follow up by attending parent training class and speaking to Dr. Tiegerman, or by speaking directly to the teacher or specialist. This gave me an opportunity to watch my child learn and challenge myself as the primary teacher at home. At times I felt like a "sponge" because there were so many different procedures that I learned by watching.

Jonathan's first friends came from his classroom at SLCD. The group of children in that class have remained friends over many years; families became much closer. There were many mornings where we all sat around the television monitor, watched and talked together. Each parent took advantage of the video system, and classroom observation became integrally involved with the school. I have often told Dr. Tiegerman that the camera in the classroom was one of the greatest gifts that she could have given parents. The opportunity to watch the classroom kept parents involved with the school and the educational process.

This chapter also discussed the long-term goals of special education which, of course, is mainstreaming. Jonathan is now in a regular elementary school class. The transitioning process from SLCD to the regular class took several years, but it was successful. I have never left SLCD because I feel that Jonathan and I can be an example to many other families who are walking this very difficult road. There were many changes in Jonathan and many changes in me, but the two of us represent a reality that early intervention works—it all started in a preschool classroom.

REFERENCES

Beckman, P., & Kohl, F. (1984). The effects of social and isolate toys on the interactions and play of integrated and nonintegrated groups of preschoolers. *Education and Training of Mentally Retarded, 19,* 169–174.

Deshler, D. D., Alley, G. R., & Carlson, S. C. (1980). Learning strategies: An approach to mainstreaming secondary students with learning disabilities. *Education Unlimited, 2,* 6–11.

Fenrick, N. J., Pearson, M. E., & Pepelnjak, J. M. (1984). The play, attending, and language of young handicapped children in integrated and segregated settings. *Journal of the Division for Early Childhood, 8,* 57–67.

Green, A., & Stoneman, Z. (1989). Attitudes of mothers and fathers of nonhandicapped children. *Journal of Early Intervention, 13,* 292–304.

Guaralnick, M. (1986). The peer relations of young handicapped and nonhandicapped children. In P. S. Strain, M. J. Guaralnick, & H. M. Walker (Eds.), *Children's social behaviors: Development, assessment, and modification* (pp. 93–140). New York: Academic Press.

Halle, J. W., Baer, D., & Spradlin, J. E. (1981). Teachers' generalized use of delay as a stimulus control procedure to increase language use in handicapped children. *Journal of Applied Behavior Analysis, 14* (4), 389–411.

Halle, J. W., Albert, C., & Anderson, S. (1984). Natural environment language assessment and intervention with severely impaired preschoolers. *Topics in Early Childhood Special Education, 4,* 36–56.

Hamblin-Wilson, C., & Thurman, S. (1990). The transition from early intervention to kindergarten: Parental satisfaction and involvement. *Journal of Early Intervention, 14,* 55–61.

Hart, B., & Risley, T. R. (1974). Using preschool materials to modify the language of disadvantaged children. *Journal of Applied Behavior Analysis, 7,* 243–256.

Hart, B., & Risley, T. R. (1975). Incidental teaching of language in the preschool. *Journal of Applied Behavior Analysis, 8,* 411–420.

Hart, B., & Risley, T. R. (1980). In vivo language training: Unanticipated and general effects. *Journal of Applied Behavior Analysis, 12,* 407–432.

Hart, B., & Risley, T. R. (1986). Incidental strategies. In R. L. Schiefelbusch (Ed.), *Language competence: Assessment and intervention.* San Diego: College Hill Press.

Hart, B., & Rogers-Warren, A. (1978). Milieu approach to teaching language. In R. L. Schiefelbusch (Ed.), *Language intervention strategies.* Baltimore: University Park Press.

McEvoy, M., Shores, R., Wehby, J., Johnson, S., & Fox, J. (1990, September). Special education teachers' implementation of procedures to promote social interaction among children in integrated settings. *Education and Training in Mental Retardation.*

McCormick, L. & Schiefelbusch, R. (1990). *Intervention processes and procedures in early language intervention.* New York: Merrill-Macmillan.

McLean, M., & Vincent, L. (1984). The use of expansions as a language intervention technique in the natural environment. *Journal of the Division for Early Childhood, 9,* 57–66.

Odom, S., Hoyson, M., Jamieson, B., & Strain, P. (1985). Increasing handicapped preschoolers peer social interactions: Cross setting and component analysis. *Journal of Applied Behavior Analysis, 18,* 3–16.

Odom, S., & McEvoy, M. (1988). Integration of young children with handicaps and normally developing children. In S. Odom and M. Karnes (Eds.), *Early intervention for infants and children with handicaps: An empirical base.* Baltimore: Paul Brooks.

Peck, C., Hayden, L., Wandschneider, M., Peterson, K., & Richarz, S. (1989). Development of integrated preschools: A qualitative inquiry into sources of resistance among parents, administrators and teachers. *Journal of Early Intervention, 13,* 353–364.

Peck, C., Richarz, S., Peterson, K., Hayden, L., Mineur, L., & Wandschneider, M. (1989). An ecological process model for implementing the LRE mandate. In R. Gaylord-Ross (Ed.), *Integration strategies for persons with handicaps* (pp. 281–297). Baltimore: Paul H. Brooks.

Raab, M., Nordquist, V., Cunningham, J., & Bleim, C. (1986). Promoting peer regard of an autistic child in a mainstream preschool using pre-enrollment activities. *Child Study Journal, 16,* 265–284.

Reichart, D., Lynch, E., Anderson, B., Svobodny, L., DiCola, J., & Mercury, M. (1989). Parental perspectives on integrated preschool opportunities for children with handicaps and children without handicaps. *Journal of Early Intervention, 13,* 6–13.

Rogers-Warren, A. K., & Warren, S. F. (1980). Pragmatics and generalization. In R. L. Schiefelbusch & J. Pickar (Eds.), *Communicative competence.* Baltimore: University Park Press.

Schaefer, E. S. (1989). Prediction of child competence from maternal beliefs and behaviors during infancy. In C. Doxiadis (Ed.), *Early influences shaping the individual* (pp. 257–268). New York: Plenum.

Shatz, M. (1982). On mechanisms of language acquisition: Can features of the communicative environment account for development? In E. Warner & L. Gleitman (Eds.), *Language acquisition: The state of the art* (pp. 102–127). New York: Cambridge University Press.

Sparling, J., & Lowman, B. (1983). Parent information needs as revealed through interests, problems, attitudes and preferences. In R. Haskins & D. Adams (Eds.), *Parent education and public policy* (pp. 304–323). Norwood, NJ: Ablex.

Warren, S. F., & Kaiser, A. P. (1988). Research in early language intervention. In S. L. Odom & M. B. Karnes (Eds.), *Early intervention for infants and children with handicaps* (pp. 89–108). Baltimore: Paul H. Brooks.

Watson, L., & Lord, C. (1982). Developing a social communication curriculum for autistic students. *Topics in Language Disorders, 3,* 1–10.

CHAPTER 8

THE SCHOOL FOR LANGUAGE AND COMMUNICATION DEVELOPMENT: THEORY, PRACTICE, AND MODEL

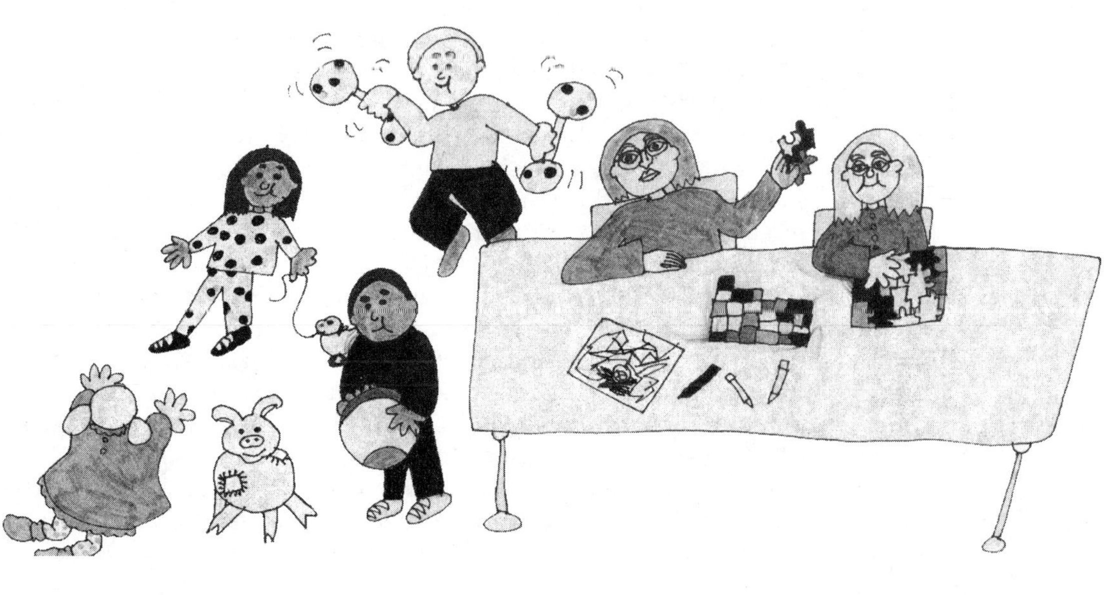

This chapter will provide students and educators with a discussion of programmatic options available for children with preschool developmental deficits. It begins with a discussion of the School for Language and Communication Development (SLCD), which I developed in July of 1985 in response to a need in Nassau County, New York. Prior to that time, the philosophy and approach described was not available in New York State in the detail and definition provided by SLCD.

The chapter describes a number of program components that are part of various schools providing services for disabled preschool children on Long Island, highlighting a number of programmatic variables: (a) program philosophy, (b) disabled population served, (c) curriculum, and (d) related services. These aspects are important in all programs and schools serving preschool children—disabled *and* nondisabled—throughout the United States. Although the chapter presents some components that make up preschool programming, in the last analysis the teacher, the therapist, the philosophy, and the service can be considered effective only if the child benefits within the framework of the program. It is with this in mind that we can begin our discussion of a model program that serves children with severe language and communication deficits.

PROGRAM PHILOSOPHY

Children with language and communication disorders present an insidious constellation of educational problems. Typically, such children during the preschool years do not present educational learning deficits other than abnormalities in language and communication behaviors. It is only over time as normal communication and language behaviors that are basic to human development and academic instruction do not develop that the child is recognized as developmentally disabled. Often, by the time this diagnosis occurs, a pattern of communication disorders has been established. The situation is further complicated by the fact that language-disordered preschool children cannot provide information and feedback concerning their needs and learning styles. Parents are often confused and frightened by children who cannot talk, cannot communicate, and cannot socialize.

The philosophy of SLCD is that the language disorder is the primary problem that must be addressed. The language disorder translates into serious learning and academic deficits during the school-age years. Because language learning provides the mechanism for all educational development, language in essence is the prerequisite program for academic acquisition and growth. The philosophy of SLCD is that the language-disordered child must be identified as early as possible in order to address language learning problems before they become instructional deficits. The school utilizes a transdisciplinary language-based learning curriculum.

Learning Domains

The transdisciplinary language program focuses on the integration of language learning by means of different modalities and different disciplinary procedures (Giangreco, York, & Rainforth, 1989). The language-disordered child is viewed across the following domain areas: cognitive, semantic, pragmatic, syntactic, phonological, social, and academic. At the preschool level the emphasis is clearly on all these areas with the exclusion of the academic. Children entering school-age programming have an additional area relating to academic-based learning instruction; there is a State Education Department academic curriculum that must be incorporated. In any case, the developmental domains represent areas of skill acquisition that provide the prerequisite underpinnings for educational growth in language and symbolic representational areas.

Population Served: Language Disordered

The children attending the School for Language and Communication Development require an intensive preschool special education experience. They range in age from three to five years and present with severe deficits in one or more of the following language areas: pragmatic, semantic, syntactic, and/or phonologic. SLCD has developed an intensive language program that provides language-disordered preschool children with a curriculum-based experience that directly relates to their individual language-learning problems. The teacher, the services, and the nature of the classroom experience are all focused on addressing each child's pragmatic, semantic, syntactic, phonological, and/or language integration learning problems.

Children with language disorders have management needs that are highly intensive and require a high degree of individualized attention and educational intervention. These children also present related developmental learning problems in areas that include perception, cognition, socialization, emotional development, and ADL (see Figure 8-1).

Programming

The School for Language and Communication Development has developed an *intensive language program* that provides language-disordered children with a smooth *transition* into the academic regimen of public school education.

Intensive language programming means that full-time language facilitation is provided in the classroom by a speech/language pathologist (SLP). In SLCD, the SLP functions as the primary service provider.

Language programming represents the central focus of the school's curriculum and model. The curriculum directly addresses the language-learning skills that are prerequisite to academic development.

Figure 8-1
The Role of Speech/Language Pathologists in the Identification, Diagnosis, and Treatment of Individuals with Cognitive-Communicative Impairments.

This document represents the cumulative effort of the members of the Committee on Language Subcommittee on Cognition and Language: Brenda Adamovich, Roberta Chapey, Patricia Larkins (ex officio), Craig Linebaugh, Marilyn Newhoff (chair), and Mark Ylvisaker under the guidance of Gilbert R. Herer, vice president for clinical affairs at the time the document was prepared and now president-elect.

Cognition and language are intrinsically and reciprocally related in both development and function. Thus, an impairment of language may disrupt one or more cognitive processes and, similarly, an impairment of one or more cognitive processes may disrupt language. Cognitively based impairments of communication are appropriately referred to as cognitive-communicative disorders and may be associated with a variety of congenital and acquired conditions in children and adults.

Certified and licensed (where applicable) speech-language pathologists are independent practitioners who are qualified to identify, diagnose, and determine the appropriateness of treatment for individuals with cognitive-communicative disorders. When treatment is indicated, speech-language pathologists develop, supervise, and/or implement a plan of treatment. Treatment of cognitive-communicative disorders has come to be included under labels such as cognitive retraining, cognitive rehabilitation, cognitive therapy, cognitive remediation, and neurotraining. Speech-language pathologists should be integral members of interdisciplinary teams engaged in the identification, diagnosis, and treatment of persons with cognitive-communicative disorders.

Source: American Speech-Language Hearing Association, Rockville Pike, Maryland

Transition means that the primary goal of programming is to appropriately remediate the language disorder so that children can return to a mainstream program. Language-disordered children require a level and a type of integrated language programming that is not provided in the public schools. Language learning is integrated into *all* academic areas by the SLP and specialists. Clinical research clearly indicates that when language disorders are appropriately addressed, the incidence of declassification increases and the severity of the disorder decreases.

Program Services

Group Services

Group Language Therapy
Group Music Therapy
Group Dance/Movement Therapy
Group Occupational Therapy
Adaptive Physical Education
Parent Training Services
Parent Language Training Class (weekly)
Peer Support Class (weekly)
Step Class (weekly)

Related Services

Individual Language Therapy
Individual Music Therapy
Individual Dance/Movement Therapy
Individual Occupational Therapy
Play Therapy

THE EDUCATIONAL MODEL

The Transdisciplinary Integrative Approach

- Transdisciplinary Integrative Educational Approach
- Speech/Language Pathologist as Primary Teacher
- Classroom as Language Laboratory
- Integrated Related Services
- Parent Language Training
- A Continuum of Educational Services
- Language Is the Primary Program for Training in Academic Areas

The School for Language and Communication Development utilizes an innovative model of transdisciplinary programming (see Figure 8-2), which requires consensus and communication among members of the professional team. Goals, activities, and interactions with children must be coordinated among specialists. The transdisciplinary model moves educational programming beyond the single-discipline approach and identifies levels of commonality across the specialty areas in terms of identification, assessment, and intervention. At SLCD the curriculum goals are generated by a transdisciplinary team of professionals; common goals are highlighted, and each specialist works on a selected activity that enhances a specific skill.

The integration of instruction across the discipline areas facilitates learning (Bailey, Simeonsson, Yoder, & Huntington, 1990). Each specialist highlights a different aspect of the skill through an activity, and as a result the language skill is reinforced through movement, through music, and through auditory training. In this respect, the transdisciplinary approach is a multimodal approach; if the child is not able to learn a skill through one form of learning, there is opportunity to acquire that skill through another form of instruction. In addition, there is always an issue concerning generalization. Learning for the language-disordered child is often context-specific and context-bound. The transdisciplinary approach allows the child to experience the use of the skill or the application of the skill by means of another modality. This increases the opportunity for language acquisition to be generalized. For the skill to be generalized, the child must learn to cross reference and cross fertilize linguistic abilities. This not only strengthens the skill, but emphasizes learning strategies.

Related Services

Another educational component at the School for Language and Communication Development is that several disciplines, such as dance movement therapy, music therapy, occupational therapy, and aural rehabilitation, can contribute

Figure 8-2
Transdisciplinary Integrative Model

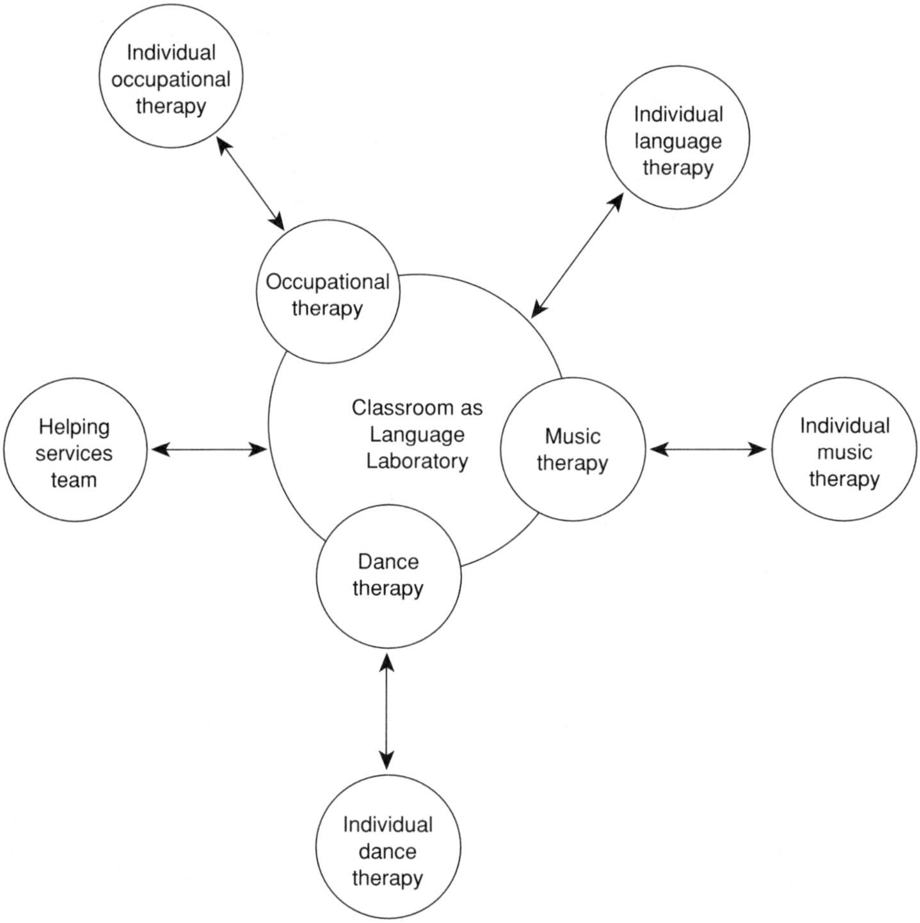

to the language-learning experience. Figure 8-2 describes the child as the central focus of programming. Each child receives a range of facilitative services, specialty areas, or related services that provide a means of enhancing the classroom language experience in a creative mode (Ploof & Feldman, 1992).

Specialists translate their educational areas into learning goals and activities that stimulate language development and communication interaction. This is consistent with the philosophy that language is a social experience and that language-disordered children require an integrated education program. This means that all of the related service specialists must be integrated into the classroom environment to provide additional opportunities to use language as a dynamic social process and to learn language by means of different disciplinary experiences.

Children are provided with group and individual therapeutic services depending on their level of developmental deficits. Children with severe deficits receive more individualized programming. As the child makes more progress, less intensive prescriptive services are needed. The goal across all of the specialty areas is to facilitate children to the point where the service can be provided in a group context. Children benefit from learning the specialty goals in a social context; they can learn in a more complex setting from peers.

The work of some of the specialists who provide services in group as well as in individual instructional settings is described in the paragraphs that follow.

The Speech/Language Pathologist

The speech/language pathologist functions as the primary classroom teacher in order to stimulate language and communication development in the classroom. The individual SLP facilitates generalization of each child's IEP goals in individual therapy and then generalizes those goals in the social context of the classroom. This means that each child receives an important application experience in the classroom; his or her language skills are generalized to a social setting of peers and adults. Pragmatic, semantic, and syntactic structures are facilitated in the classroom by getting children to communicate with each other, take turns, respond to questions, initiate topics and information, and participate in activities. It is the responsibility of the classroom SLP to interface directly with all of the specialists.

The classroom SLP serves as the head of the transdisciplinary classroom team, which consists of the speech/language pathologist, the occupational therapist, the dance movement therapist, the aural rehabilitation specialist, the music therapist, the psychologist, and the individual speech/language pathologist. The team meets on a weekly basis to discuss the goals related to each child, the child's IEP, the child's progress, and specific activities/lesson plans that should be generated to facilitate the child's language development at any given stage of development. This allows each member of the transdisciplinary team an opportunity to discuss the child's progress across the specialty areas on an ongoing basis. It also allows each member of the team to fine-tune goals and activities for each child on his or her case load.

Each of the related service professionals translates his or her area of expertise into specific goals that correspond to the language development goals generated by the speech/language pathologist and implemented in the classroom, such as:

1. Child will maintain appropriate eye gaze with an adult.
2. Child will demonstrate appropriate nonverbal turn-taking behaviors.
3. Child will request objects from an adult through verbalization.
4. Child will respond appropriately to one step verbal directions.
5. Child will encode utterances utilizing a mean length of utterance of two.

These goals are cross referenced across all of the specialty areas. The sections that follow explain how they are translated into each educational-therapeutic area.

The Occupational Therapist

Occupational therapy involves any activity in which one engages for evaluation, diagnosis, and treatment of problems interfering with functional performance in persons impaired by physical illness or injury, emotional disorders, congenital or developmental disability, or the aging process in order to achieve optimum functioning and for prevention and health maintenance (Hanft & Humphry, 1989). Specific occupational therapy services include, but are not limited to, activities of daily living (ADL); the design, fabrication, and application of splints; sensorimotor activities, the use of specifically designed crafts; guidance in the selection and use of adaptive equipment; therapeutic activities to enhance functional performance; prevocational evaluation and training; and consultation concerning the adaptation of physical environments for the disabled. These services are provided to individuals or groups through medical, health, educational, and social systems (American Occupational Therapy Association, April 18, 1977).

Occupational therapy in an educational setting for language-disordered children may be provided on an individual or a classroom consultation basis. It is the intent of the occupational therapist to treat the whole child to perform essential preschool and school-age tasks (Hopkins, 1988).

An occupational therapy evaluation encompasses gross motor skills, fine motor skills, sensory functioning, cognitive skills, perceptual skills, visual motor skills, and personal-social skills.

Gross motor skills involve the child's ability to move through space with regard to accomplishment and quality of movement. Balance and equilibrium reactions, reflex integration, ball handling, ascending and descending stairs, and developmental motor milestones may be within a child's ability to maintain an upright sitting position. Fine motor skills take into account hand development—reciprocal, assistive, and bilateral usage. In the academic setting, writing skills are a major concern. Sensory functioning requires the input of a stimulus for processing and output via an adaptive response. The sensory input may be auditory, visual, gustatory, tactile, proprioceptive, kinesthetic, or vestibular (Wilbarger, 1984). Cognitive skills include age-level acquired knowledge in reference to color, shape, or size recognition, knowledge of the alphabet and numbers, and relatedness to toys/objects in the environment. Examples of perceptual skills involve nonmotor abilities to use figure ground, spatial relations, sequential memory, visual closure, form constancy, visual memory, and visual discrimination. Visual-motor skills involve the ability for the hand to perform what the brain perceives and the ability for the brain to perceive what the hand needs to perform. During formal testing a child copies a variety of lines and shapes; printing is an academic related visual motor skill. Personal social skills include activities of daily living and the ability to perform developmentally appropriate self-care skills required in an academic setting. This may include dressing activities and the ability to put on and take off outerwear and to manipulate buttons, zippers, fasteners, laces, and shoes. In the classroom, the student may be expected to manage his or her own lunchbox, toilet independently, and assist in classroom cleanup.

Treatment intervention typically follows a developmentally based sensorimotor approach (Anderson, 1986). A remedial approach may be utilized to teach a splinter skill to a child in order to meet expectations with peers, e.g., tying shoes. A sensory integrative approach is based on the premise that development occurs as the result of organization of vestibular, tactile, and proprioceptive information. Development will occur as a functional intervention in the areas of reflex maturation, body schema, postural control, balance and equilibrium reactions, and bilateral integration. These sensorimotor activities in turn develop perceptual skills such as body coordination in skipping and descending stairs and eye-hand coordination in lacing and printing. Auditory language skills may be developed by facilitating the ability of the body to organize sensory input. The occupational therapist attempts to provide the child with an opportunity to stimulate lower-level neurological reactions that will affect higher-level language skills.

The OT uses knowledge of physical, social, and emotional functions to determine the motor developmental needs of a specific child and group. The therapist then identifies a program of activity leading to the development of fine motor skills (Williamson, 1988). The skills learned may be as basic as the daily living tasks of bathing, dressing, and eating, or they may be as sophisticated as the complex grapho-motor skills of letter writing or figure drawing. The following occupational therapy goals relate to the above-mentioned language goals and include appropriate activities that facilitate learning.

1. Draw a Design

This activity may involve visual, perceptual, motor, and sensory skills. The task may involve different mediums such as paper/pencil, brush/paint, shaving cream, or clay. Three-dimensional designs can be made with popsicle sticks or straws.

The activity may be graded by having the child imitate a design or, on a higher level, copy a design. In the first instance, the child has a demonstration and visual cuing. The ability to copy means the item is presented and the child draws without demonstration.

This activity may follow a developmental sequence beginning with random drawing and progressing to vertical, horizontal, circular, and intersecting lines, and square and triangle shapes. Regard to boundaries may also be considered as well as expansion of the activity by considering the combination of designs to make a picture, coloring within designated space, and hand grasp.

During verbal directions a child's eye gaze should be maintained. Turn-taking during design construction may be structured for sharing objects and for nonverbal interaction with peers. If a specific item is needed, the child may be prompted "want more" or "give me crayon." If the therapist wants to provide an opportunity for the child to respond appropriately to a one-step verbal direction, an array of choices are available: "pick up pencil," "draw here," "make a circle." The child may describe the picture—"that's a house," "that's me"—to utilize productive language skills.

2. Pinching

In order to use our own "pinchers" of thumb and index finger, objects such as clothespins or blunt tweezers may be utilized to manipulate clay, small beads, and coins. This activity may be set up as a tabletop task or as the child sits straddled over a roll to facilitate midline crossing, trunk rotation, and visual tracking. An array of cognitive skills may be emphasized including color, size, and shape discrimination. The pinching game will facilitate hand development and proximal stability for distal motor control. The command to "take peg" facilitates eye gaze with adults and following one-step verbal commands. Turn-taking may be set up with the child taking a peg, then the therapist taking a peg in sequence, establishing a routine. If pegs are positioned out of the child's reach, or set up so as to require more pegs, facilitation of the child's requesting the object can be met. The child may request "want blue," "want more," or "I do" throughout the session.

3. The Swing

The swing provides movement experiences. A child may be placed on the platform in a prone position to encourage development of the extensor muscle groups. Trunk extension is required for maintaining an upright sitting posture. The therapist may ask the child to look at her face and take an object such as a beanbag from her hand, then to throw the bean bag at a designated target. When the child completes the task, he may be encouraged to verbalize "I do," "I hit it."

4. Manipulatives, e.g., Legos, Tinkertoys

The child is presented with interlocking toys that require bilateral motor coordination, reciprocal and assistive hand usage, and visual motor and visual perceptual skills. The ability to interlock toys can be used to encourage eye gaze by having the child seated opposite with the therapist holding the block and saying, "I build." Turn-taking is facilitated by offering the block and directing the child "you do." With completion of the task, the child may spontaneously be prompted to describe the structure.

Credit: Vera Gallagher, OTR Specialist, School for Language and Communication Development

The Dance Movement Therapist

Dance therapy is defined as the psychotherapeutic use of movement as a process that furthers the emotional and physical integration of the individual.

Social, emotional, cognitive, and physical problems are dealt with through intervention on a body movement level (Levy, 1988). At the School for Language and Communication Development, dance therapy is provided as part of a transdisciplinary approach; it serves as a creative stimulus for expression and for imaginative exploration of interaction with the environment.

In addition to the development of motor abilities, such as running, jumping, and leaping, dance therapy is involved with self-expression, authentic communication, and the pure joy of moving (Ekstein, 1983). In addition, the dance therapist is concerned with the quality of motor skills development and the acquisition of those skills based on the integration of the fundamental areas of body awareness, body image, spatial awareness, rhythmic response, and coordination. The quality of interaction between the child and his classmates and the adults in his environment, is also carefully monitored. Body movement, communication, and relatedness are interconnected; dance therapy addresses all three at once.

Movement is a basic and very important function of life. This is most apparent in the early years when children are naturally tuned into their bodies and when they learn by doing. During this period, they are also learning about the body and emotional responses to the environment. For example, a child's body receives a lot of attention during feeding, dressing, toileting, and other activities of daily living. They are also learning about how their behavior is being accepted by parents and other significant adults. Children view many activities in terms of how they feel. The excitement of an activity and the joy in performing it or in successfully achieving it give the child important positive reinforcement for his performances. Action is experienced on a body level, then becomes translated into self-esteem, self-confidence, and ultimately motivation to learn. It cannot be stressed enough how important positive self-regard and self-esteem are in the ability to communicate effectively.

The dance therapist can provide important experiences that will nurture healthy body attitude, develop a particular motor ability, and, at the same time, be a lot of fun. Going up a climber and sliding down a slide to the cheering of teacher and classmates can be fulfilling to any child. Moving around in a circle, holding hands with classmates, and enjoying the rhythm of music can develop a sense of acceptance and belonging. Being given the opportunity to move freely or to improvise a dance can develop independence and creative expression.

Credit: Sarah Becker, ADTR Specialist, School for Language and Communication Development

The benefits of dance therapy in early intervention are extraordinary as learning occurs on a body level. From infancy, a child learns about herself, others, and her environment through her body as she employs her five senses (Stern, 1985). Prior to the development of formalized language, she learns to express herself nonverbally. She communicates by crying, smiling, laughing, and eventually gesturing—all before she has the ability to speak. Young children are motivated by movement and receive instant physical gratification through the pleasure experienced during motor activity. The needs of the whole child are addressed in the natural, familiar context of movement games. As the child moves, she incorporates knowledge of herself, others, and her environment into her learning experience.

Dance therapy is a viable tool to be used in an educational setting for language-disordered children. This multisensory approach to motor development helps to integrate nonverbal and verbal communication with physical coordination, motor planning and sequencing, body tension, spatial awareness, and rhythmic ability (Greenspan & Pollock, 1989). Language aspects, such as pragmatic deficits, disfluency, apraxia, and syntactic errors, are frequently related to the motor areas listed above. Pragmatic deficits, such as interacting with one's environment, may be related to spatial awareness; disfluency may be related to upper body tension and limited rhythmic ability; apraxia and syntax may be related to motor planning and sequencing. The interrelationship between symbolic language and motor aspects is undeniable; a motor-oriented intervention should be used to facilitate maximum success for young children.

The dance movement therapist develops a program of prescriptive treatment to facilitate acquisition of motor skills in individual as well as group sessions. The following dance movement therapy activities relate to the above-mentioned language goals.

1. "Hello" Song

The child sits facing the therapist as the group sings a "hello" song. The child's and the therapist's names will be incorporated into the song. (Address goals 1 and 2.)

2. Rhythmic Body Part Tapping

The child and the therapist take turns as leader and follower during body part tapping exercises. The therapist elicits movement suggestions from the child. (Address goals 2, 4, and 5.)

3. Gross Motor Obstacle Course Activity

The child engages in an obstacle course activity, incorporating prepositional concepts *(in, out, up, down, under)*. The child also encodes actions (e.g., "go in", "go on," etc). (Address goals 2, 4, and 5.).

4. Relaxation Activity

The child requests hand lotion to rub on body periphery (hands, arms, and face) to promote relaxation and the development of body boundaries. (Address goals 3, 4, and 5.)

5. "Good-Bye" Song

The child faces the therapist to sing good-bye, in same manner as "hello" song. (Address goals 1 and 2.)

Credit: Nancy Sheehan, ADTR Specialist, School for Language and Communication Development

The Music Therapist

The music therapist uses music as a primary modality in treating children with language and communication disorders. She uses her expertise to facilitate auditory processing skills. There are aspects of speech that are similar to aspects of music, such as rhythm, patterning, volume, pitch, and prosody. These aspects of music are used to facilitate verbal and social interaction in children (Alvin, 1975). According to Nordoff and Robbins (1971) *music* might be defined as experiences of rhythmic and tonal variety. These experiences relate to all aspects of an individual and how he or she views the world—to body movement and dance, to one's emotional life, to communication and thought, and to speech and language.

Just as all human beings have an inborn capacity for learning language, they also have the innate capability of responding to music. It is no coincidence that the five basic elements of music—rhythm, pitch, dynamics, pulse, and form—are intimately connected with the production of speech. Thus, music has a unique role to play in our work with language-disordered children (Bruscia, 1989).

Spoken language is both rhythmic and melodic. Each sentence has a rhythmic form, stress patterns, and variations in pitch and inflection that help to communicate its meaning. Through both singing and instrumental work, the language-disordered child can move toward greater language proficiency. The music therapist must be skilled at adapting conventional materials and finding other appropriate materials for use with children who have difficulty in the processing and expression of language (Alvin, 1976). Singing, which is a natural musical activity for preschool children, aims toward improving auditory perception, processing, and memory; voice quality, production of speech sounds; learning and retention of language; and production of meaningful communication. Songs with suitable subjects, actions, tempo, mood, and word setting can enhance the linguistic, perceptual, and cognitive goals set by the classroom teacher.

An activity may be introduced in several sensory modalities to make the experience more holistic and to reinforce learning on many different levels (Nordoff & Robbins, 1971). Eventually, visual and kinesthetic input may be reduced in order to strengthen the child's auditory mode. For example, when exploring ranges of pitch, the child may be asked to move his body up and down, corresponding to high and low pitches, while following a model or blackboard diagram.

The music therapist utilizes the qualities of music and relates those qualities to language. She uses a wide variety of techniques and activities, including free singing, song singing, rhythmic work, instrumental work, and action songs, all aimed at teaching and reinforcing the acquisition of language. Music therapy also teaches basic vocabulary, as well as helping the child achieve the difficult task of sequencing an event. It encourages creativity and vocal play, which can help the child achieve the vocal confidence and skill needed to become an effective language initiator (Boxhill, 1985).

In music therapy, children use rhythm instruments, objects in the classroom, and their voices to create mood and action. In creating a thunderstorm, for example, the activity begins with the calm stillness before the storm. The excitement and activity of the storm is created by the instruments that build a dramatic crescendo in the activity. When the storm subsides, the instruments are played more softly. The vocabulary emphasized include: *storm, cloud, start, stop, rain, lightning, thunder, loud,* and *soft*. At the conclusion of the music activity, it is clear that the children share the satisfaction of having made a personal contribution to the larger group experience. "Music therapy is a systematic process of intervention wherein the therapist helps the client to achieve health using musical experiences and the relationships that develop through them as dynamic forces of change" (Bruscia, 1989).

There are two separate and distinct aspects of the music therapy program at SLCD:

1. Using music as a means to reinforce language goals, based on the close connection between music and speech. For example:

   (a) repetitive singing and chanting aids fluency; (b) word substitution songs help build vocabulary and organize thinking in terms of categories, associations, etc.; (c) leaving out a word or phrase when singing a familiar song assists with word-finding; (d) learning a song in its entirety promotes auditory memory and sequencing skills; (e) singing call-and-response songs gives children practice in the turn-taking needed in conversation.

2. Using music as an alternate mode of communication, since music is nonverbal communication. A basic principle of music therapy is the concept of the "music child" (Nordoff & Robbins, 1971), which includes the ability to respond to music that exists in every human being. Music can cut right through a person's pathology or disability and reach the music child, the part of an individual that is healthy. By nurturing the music child, the borders of the personality can be expanded and a new and richer self can emerge through (a) the establishment or reestablishment of interpersonal relationships; (b) the bringing about of self-esteem through self-actualization; and (c) the utilization of the unique potential of rhythm to energize and bring order. The creative process of using music to facilitate language development is used as a primary experience with language-disordered children.

The following music therapy activities relate to the above- mentioned language goals.

1. Greeting: Contact Song

A greeting song that incorporates the child's name is improvised. This becomes the child's "contact song," and is repeated each week. The song helps the child become oriented to the situation and, through repetition, simple phrases are learned (for example: "Hello, Jimmy, it's time for music"). The therapist seeks to establish eye contact, and pauses to allow time for the child to respond both verbally and nonverbally.

2. Introducing a Simple Structure Using Movements "to the Music"
The child follows song commands such as "clap your hands to the music." The child verbally requests a movement when given a choice (for example, "should we clap or stamp?"). The child performs verbal closure when therapist omits a word (for example, "clap your _____ to the music").

3. Instrumental Improvisation
The child selects an instrument he or she wishes to play. The therapist provides accompaniment; they take turns leading and following changes in tempo and volume.

4. "Five Little Fingers" (by Carol Robbins)
In this song, the child counts his fingers and points to appropriate body parts. The child takes initiative and chooses which body part to sing about next.

5. "Good-bye" Song
Closure is provided by a "good-bye" song, again using the child's name and stating "it's time to say good-bye." The child and therapist take turns strumming a guitar and saying "good bye."

Credit: Jackie Levin, MTR Specialist, School for Language and Communication Development

Aural Rehabilitation Specialist

The aural rehabilitation specialist works at facilitating the relationship between auditory awareness and language development. Children who appear to present with a lack of auditory awareness receive intensive training in sound stimulation, sound facilitation, auditory enhancement, and auditory integration (Gillet, 1993). Children with perceptual and central auditory processing problems such as hearing impairment and autism receive intensive instruction by the aural rehabilitation specialist.

Auditory training is a method for increasing the use of the auditory channel in concept development and language learning. The primary goal is to develop listening skills at an early stage in life, from birth to five years of age (Northcott, 1984). At SLCD, listening has to be learned. A child with a language and communication disorder must be taught first to be aware of sound, to discriminate among various sounds, to attach meaning to them, and then to localize or tell from which direction the sound is coming. Four major classifications of sound are used in learning to listen: gross sounds, environmental sounds, music, and speech. These are developed simultaneously, not separately.

Listening goes on all during the child's day. Therefore, attention is called to gross sounds, even during structured activities, to various environmental sounds as they occur naturally, to the music on the stereo or radio, as well as calling to and talking to the child about what is happening. It is essential for the child to develop an auditory feedback system comprised of audition, auditory memory, auditory sequencing, and monitoring of his own voice (Lowell & Stoner, 1960). To develop this system, the child's language, cognitive skills, and listening must be simultaneously encouraged. The child must recognize the sounds he makes and those made by others. He is encouraged to vocalize in response to adult models. He is also encouraged to babble, to imitate single words, and to respond to inflectional and temporal patterns. He is gradually expected to remember increasingly longer phrases and then sentence patterns, first in imitation and then spontaneously.

The following aural rehabilitation activities relate to the above-mentioned language goals.

1. "Loud Drum/Soft Drum"
The child marches to the loud drum, and tiptoes to the soft drum.

2. "Rocking Horse"
The child listens to the music of the Rocking Horse; he moves when he hears the music and stops when the music stops.

3. "Find the Bell"
The child finds the bell by localizing the sound in the immediate environment.

4. "Wake Up/Go to Sleep"
The child plays at waking up when he hears the alarm clark and going to sleep when it stops.

Credit: Lynn Senko, Teacher of the Deaf Specialist, School for Language and Communication Development

The School Psychologist

The overall task of school psychologists is to identify specific needs of children through ongoing diagnostic evaluations and classroom consultations (Salvia & Ysseldyke, 1991). They use a holistic approach and play a major role in solving classroom-related problems. They work with the teacher in the classroom to help in developing and implementing behavior-management programs.

In a central-based program with severely language-disordered children, the school psychologist plays an integrative role. He or she participates in the daily functioning of the classroom, and, in addition, functions as a liaison between the school and the home setting. The school psychologist provides direct intervention to children and parents, provides individual and group play therapy, assists families in crisis intervention, and monitors children's individual cognitive progress.

The underlying policy concerning behavioral management is that as children learn language, they more effectively and appropriately regulate their own behavior and the behavior of other social interactants.

Language-disordered children can *only* learn about social behaviors, language rules, and the social use of language in a social context. Language learning is in fact a social learning process. The social bases of normal language development emphasize the need to provide social learning contexts for language-disordered children. The social learning environment of the classroom provides a normalizing experience. Social learning provides these children with the opportunity to use their language skills and behaviors to regulate the environment in more socially appropriate ways. The language-disordered child who tantrums, screams, and self-stimulates needs to be involved in an activity that will provide the opportunity to communicate his or her true intentions, hence, activities should foster language stimulation and enhancement.

When children learn that there is a contingency relationship between their behavior and their environment, inappropriate behaviors decrease. A variety of social procedures are used to teach and reinforce appropriate interactional behaviors. Modeling and imitation procedures along with differential reinforcement of other behaviors (DRO) are utilized to systematically shape social behaviors. Primary reinforcers, tokens, and social reinforcers are used in context to shape and maintain appropriate classroom behaviors. The most important aspect to social training is consistency in environmental contingency and training across teachers, parents, and adults.

Parents and teachers are trained to use the behavioral procedures described during parent-training and staff-training sessions (Baker, 1984). Parents must agree to all behavioral procedures and participate in the child's training (Wright, Granger, & Sameroff, 1984). The variety of educational contexts provides a mechanism for generalization of behaviors. Finally, children and staff are closely monitored by the transdisciplinary team to determine the effectiveness of all teaching procedures; data recording and analysis validate child performance changes.

Many of the language goals generated by the curriculum team have direct correlation to the goals of the psychologist as a classroom consultant. The psychologist works closely with the classroom speech pathologist to develop and implement management goals, interactional goals, developmental play goals, and self-concept goals (Sattler, 1988). For example, in helping the child demonstrate appropriate turn-taking behaviors, the psychologist in conjunction with the teacher may develop a behavioral system that fosters self-regulatory behaviors in social contexts. At the same time, the child is learning the language necessary to request and regulate his own behaviors and others'; he is also being rewarded for this behavior through the use of a structured positive reinforcement program. Thus, appropriate modeling and teaching coupled with a behavioral approach leads to a child who communicates successfully and appropriately.

Another goal that the psychologist may have for an individual child or the entire class is to develop an ability to identify and to express emotions appropriately. A child with a language and communication disorder is often a child with a sense of failure, low self-esteem, and poor frustration tolerance. She cannot communicate her needs to others and will develop inappropriate ways to express these frustrations through anger and rage. Asking such a child to request objects from an adult through verbalizations not only addresses her expressive language but also focuses on the inner child. The speech pathologist, with the input of the psychologist, is providing a way for the child to have success by enabling her to communicate these emotions appropriately via language. The psychologist recommends activities geared toward building self-esteem in the classroom; individual play therapy also can address these issues on an individual basis (Reynolds & Gutkin, 1982).

Credit: Dr. Helene Mermelstein, Psy.D., Chief Psychologist, School for Language and Communication Development

PROGRAMMATIC COMPONENTS

The New Classroom Teacher

Since all the children at SLCD present with severe language and communication deficits, a primary philosophy component has to do with the type of teacher in the classroom. Historically, in New York State, the speech/language pathologist functioned on an itinerant basis, providing pull-out related services in special-education classrooms. At SLCD, the related service became the primary service, and the speech/language pathologist became the primary classroom teacher. Although SLPs are uniquely trained to deal with the language-disordered population, it was initially very difficult for an SLP who had been trained in an academic setting with practicum experience in individual therapy to transition into the classroom. Special-education teachers are trained in the development of classroom-based instruction as well as in group analysis and group management. It became a challenge in staff development programming to develop a set of classroom-based instructional skills for the speech/language pathologist.

If SLPs are going to function as preschool teachers in the future, the nature of academic instruction must be changed to include this new professional responsibility. The SLP has always provided services outside the classroom. The experiences at SLCD support the role of the SLP as a primary classroom teacher; however, it is clear that several additional courses and practical experiences are necessary at the university level.

No other professional has the SLP's expertise in facilitating language-learning skills in developmentally disordered children. The success of SLCD can be attributed to the quality of the language-based instruction provided to children. Having an SLP as a teacher presents the language-disordered child with the opportunity for an immersion language experience.

Regulated Services

An important issue at SLCD was the fact that each language-disordered child required not only a social group learning experience but also an individual learning experience. There are many children who are so severely impaired that the nature of the instruction must be highly individualized since the group does not provide educational benefit. As a result, the services, as well as the group size, need to be regulated to the child's level of functioning. The rule of thumb at SLCD has been (a) the more severely language disordered the child, the smaller the group size (the smaller the instructional class) must be, and (b) the more severely language disordered the child, the more individualized the related therapeutic services must be. As the child's language ability improves and increases, the size of the class gets larger and the related services shift from individualized to group-based instruction.

Some preschool programs have the flexibility to provide individualized instruction across a number of therapeutic specialty areas (Deal, Dunst, & Trivette, 1989; Dunst, Johanson, Trivette, & Hamby, 1991). In this way, the quantitative as well as the qualitative learning needs of the child can be addressed. Language-disordered children exhibit highly individualized learning problems and learning styles. It is important that the educational environment identify these idiosyncratic aspects and develop learning programs that facilitate the child's individual style of language learning.

It is the philosophy of SLCD that the language-disordered child must be gradually integrated into a larger, more complex, more demanding social environment. It is, therefore, important to understand the prescriptive nature of the child's language deficit. Figure 8-3 shows the changing IEP recommendations for Bryan as he progressed over a three-year period. Note that as his language abilities increased, programming shifted from individual to group-based learning experiences.

Educational Continuum of Services

In 1975, with the passage of Public Law 94-142, Education of All Handicapped Children Act (EAHCA), disabled children ages five to twenty-one were mandated a free and appropriate public education (see Chapter 4). In the years following the passage of this bill, it became clear that children below the age of five who were disabled also needed services. In 1986, Public Law 99-457 extended the rights and privileges mandated in the earlier bill to preschoolers aged three to

Figure 8-3
IEP Recommendations for Bryan, 1988–1990

IEP 1988

Child's Name:	Bryan Smith	
Date of Birth:	1/1/85	
Placement:	School for Language and Communication Development	
Class Ratio:	12:2:2	
Primary Teacher:	Speech/Language Pathologist	
Related Services:	Occupational Therapy:	Individual instruction 2 times a week
	Dance Movement Therapy:	Individual instruction 2 times a week; 4 times a week, group
	Auditory Training:	Individual 2 times a week; 2 times a week, group

IEP 1989

Child's Name:	Bryan Smith	
Date of Birth:	1/1/85	
Placement:	School for Language and Communication Development	
Class Ratio:	12:1:1	
Primary Teacher:	Speech/Language Pathologist	
Related Services:	Occupational Therapy:	Individual instruction 2 times a week
	Dance Movement Therapy:	Group, 4 times a week
	Auditory Training:	Group, 2 times a week
	Music Therapy:	Group, 2 times a week

IEP 1990

Child's Name:	Bryan Smith	
Date of Birth:	1/1/85	
Placement:	School for Language and Communication Development	
Class Ratio:	15:1:1	
Primary Teacher:	Speech/Language Pathologist	
Related Services:	Occupational Therapy:	Individual, 1 time a week
	Dance Movement Therapy:	Group, 1 time a week
	Auditory Training:	Group, 1 time a week
	Music Therapy:	Group, 1 time a week

five years. This established a continuum of services that guarantees educational support for the family and for the disabled person until adulthood.

Public Law 99-457 stresses the significance and importance of early identification and early intervention; it also fills a gap in the educational life of the child. Once diagnosed, the disabling condition needs to be addressed. It is problematic to identify a problem at age three and not be able to provide educational programming until age five. Clearly, programming must be available early and must continue to be available for as long as the child needs the service (Hains, Rosenkoetter, & Fowler, 1991).

The passage of these two bills allowed for the development of a comprehensive network system of programs throughout the United States. A family traveling with a disabled child from New York to California would be ensured of a program wherever they stopped along the way. It also created a regulatory system to ensure the quality of programs by establishing standards of education for the disabled. These educational standards are obviously very important in regulating programs, certifying teachers, and establishing minimum standards of educational curricula and programming. These two bills recognize the rights of the disabled to achieve their potential and also acknowledge society's responsibility in its commitment. Educational entitlement ensures that from federal to state to local governmental levels, programs for the disabled will be provided in schools.

PRESCHOOL PROGRAMS

Early intervention programs can incorporate many educational variables. New York State has a multitude of early intervention programs that serve different populations of preschool children with disabilities and have different philosophies and educational curricula. Although it is difficult to compare and contrast these various programs, their inherent programmatic variables are presented for discussion and analysis. The sections that follow point out a number of variables that can be utilized by teachers and parents to evaluate program effectiveness for a specific child (Tingey, 1989).

1. Philosophical Approach

Without a doubt, it is the philosophical orientation of the program that determines the early intervention model. Underlying all programmatic compounds is the program's philosophy, which includes methodology, teaching approach, services, and classroom-based instruction. It is important for teachers and parents to be clear about the program's philosophy and to understand how that philosophy filters into or extends into educational instruction for the language-disordered preschool child.

An example of programmatic philosophy is described by the Association for Children with Learning Disabilities (ACLD): The ACLD Early Intervention Program has been established to meet the needs of infants and young children with developmental disabilities and their families. In order to succeed in this task, basic philosophical guidelines have been established which provide the programming for the program's ongoing growth and development. ACLD's Early Intervention Program has created an individualized program that assesses and intervenes in each child's development for the purpose of helping them reach their fullest potential. In order to achieve this end, a transdisciplinary approach to educational and therapeutic services has been established.

Simply stated, the philosophy of ACLD involves the approach that family and staff can together develop holistic educational/therapeutic goals and objectives. These goals and objectives are worked on by all staff members and are reinforced by parents at home. Each staff member assumes responsibility for communicating the nature, purpose, and means of achieving these goals to parents.

2. Educational Setting

Many programs are center-based, which means that the child attends the school for a specific number of hours during the course of the day or week; some programs provide home-based instruction as well. When the services incorporate nondisabled children, they are referred to as integrated or inclusionary. When a program educates only disabled children the setting is referred to as self-contained. The trend today is to develop inclusion-based programs that educate children with disabilities along with normal children. Some center-based special education programs affiliate with day care or nursery school programs so that disabled preschool children receive therapeutic programming in an educational environment in the morning with other disabled children and socialization in a day care program in the afternoon with nondisabled children.

The Little Village School Early Intervention Program provides developmentally delayed infants and their families with comprehensive services. The program provides multiple settings for ongoing, positive relationships as a function of the children's developmental needs. The school- or center-based program involves parents and children participating in three-hour training sessions twice a week at the Little Village School. The home-based program involves the parents and children participating in an educational and therapeutic program in the home, which is based on the child's individual needs and may include occupational therapy, physical therapy, and speech therapy. At the Little Village School, children may receive center-based programming only, home-based programming only, or some combination of the two.

3. Types and Intensity of Service Provision

Each educational program provides different types of therapeutic services depending on the type of disabled population that is being served. How often services are provided, the duration of each therapeutic session, and the goals related to instruction are all linked to the philosophical orientation of the program. Some programs for physically challenged children may provide physical therapy five times a week. Some programs such as SLCD, which serves severely language-disordered children, may not offer physical therapy at all, but provide language and communication services five times a week. Therapeutic services represent a programmatic menu. Each program individualizes therapeutic services as a function of the child's developmental and clinical needs. The child's Individual Education Plan (IEP) is generated by an interdisciplinary team and specifies the type of therapeutic service along with the number of times the service is provided during the course of a week.

St. Charles Preschool Program serves children who are multiply disabled. St. Charles provides physical therapy, music therapy, bilingual programming, speech and language therapy, special education services, psychological services, social work, occupational therapy, neurodevelopmental assessment, and many other medical services.

4. Disabling Conditions

The type of child and the nature of the disabling condition determine the kind of program and therapeutic intervention provided by the program. Children with different problems require different services, different teachers, and different types of educational curricula and instruction. It is important for parents and teachers to understand the specific developmental needs of various disabled populations in order to individualize programming for each child.

The St. Charles Preschool Program serves children with disabling conditions that include cerebral palsy; spina bifida; respiratory, neurological, and orthopedic problems; congenital abnormalities and disabilities; mental retardation; severe speech and language delay; and developmental disability.

The North Shore University Hospital-Preschool Division provides services to children with primary language disorders and other associated developmental problems. This program does not provide services to children who are primarily mentally retarded, emotionally disturbed, or hearing impaired, since these needs are met by other agencies in the community. The North Shore Preschool Program has a language-oriented curriculum that is integrated into all aspects of the program. The Preschool Development Program provides a setting for learning and growing, for the development of interest in people, ideas, and things, for the acquisition and strengthening of skills, and for the remediation of areas of language dysfunction.

5. Staffing

The type of staff necessary for an early intervention program depends on the nature of the population being served and the philosophy of the program. Whether the services should be provided by certified, noncertified, or paraprofessional staff is often determined by the professional disciplines themselves or state education department requirements. The critical issue in terms of staffing relates to how the staff interfaces across discipline areas on a programmatic level. Is the program interdisciplinary or transdisciplinary? Do staff members meet on a daily basis or a monthly basis? Are there staff development opportunities in the program? Are staff members encouraged to get master's degrees and/or doctoral degrees? Without a doubt, the quality of the program is significantly related to the professional level of the staff.

The Early Intervention Program at the Little Village School creates an initial positive bond between families of children with disabling conditions and the professionals with whom they are involved. This early relationship provides the basic relationship for future learning. The coordinated services of the therapeutic and educational specialists provide experiences that enable the parent, who is the primary deliverer of services to the child, to receive maximum assistance in becoming a confident nurturer. The Little Village School's medical director is responsible for coordinating the multidisciplinary team's services. The team is comprised of a speech/language therapist, a special education teacher, a physical therapist, an occupational therapist, a movement therapist, a nurse, a social worker, and a psychologist. Close involvement of the staff provides guidance and support for siblings, parents, and interfamily relationships. Each professional's expertise is shared with parents during therapy and during educational sessions. The child's initial assessment conferences and re-evaluation conferences are scheduled three times a year with parents. The team also facilitates and coordinates the services of other outside agencies that may be involved with the family. When a child is ready to leave the Early Intervention Program, the entire staff is involved in assisting the parents to select the most beneficial treatment facility for that child.

6. Family Involvement

Public Law 99-457 mandates that early intervention programs should be family-focused and family-oriented. There is a great deal of difference among programs about defining what constitutes family involvement. Should parents function as teachers? Should there be formal parent training? Should parents be involved with classrooms on a daily basis? Should parents make educational decisions? Should parents be voting members of committees on preschool special education? How should parents be involved in the educational planning for their child? Various programs provide different levels of family involvement.

At SLCD, parents are integral members of the team. They are their children's primary educators and are involved on all levels of planning as well as in implementing the children's programs. Families are encouraged to be actively involved in the ongoing development of their children and the activities of the Early Intervention Program at the Association for Children with Learning Disabilities. This active involvement is facilitated through the formation of social-emotional support groups and parent workshops. Participation in the educational and therapeutic process is strongly encouraged by having parents directly involved in classroom and home activities. The program seeks new ways to evaluate parent-child interactions for the purpose of assisting parents to become more active in their child's developmental process. The key to this process is communication between the program and the families.

7. *The Evaluation Process*

In order to determine whether or not the child has a disabling problem, he or she needs to be evaluated by an educational team of professionals. The kind of evaluations and the members of the professional team are often a function of the program's philosophy. The definition of a comprehensive evaluation and what constitutes a comprehensive evaluation varies from program to program and from state to state.

In order to identify the appropriate program, a comprehensive evaluation must be performed and recommendations must be generated by the educational team. Whether the program utilizes an interdisciplinary or transdisciplinary approach is also a function of the program's philosophy. The final step in programmatic decision making involves the generation of an Individualized Education Plan (IEP) that will detail goals and services for a specific child. Again, the number and type of professionals constituting the educational team, the types of evaluation tools utilized, and the nature of the decision-making process are all related to program philosophy and state requirements.

At St. Charles Preschool Program, children are evaluated by an interdisciplinary team that includes professionals trained in developmental pediatrics, orthopedics, clinical psychology, social work, speech/language pathology, occupational therapy, physical therapy, educational therapy, educational diagnostics, and any other specialty required, e.g., cardiology and/or neurology. After the evaluations are completed, the team makes recommendations for educational placement and therapeutic services. An Individual Education Plan is written by the team and families are an integral part of the team approach. The child is then placed in a special-education class; educational instruction is provided by a certified special-education teacher and teacher aide. All therapy is provided on a one-on-one basis by certified and licensed professionals. The treatment team meets regularly to share information that is an integral part of the child's rehabilitation.

This is not meant to be an exhaustive list of programmatic variables. It includes only some of the variables that can be utilized by parents and teachers to determine appropriate placement for preschool child with language disorders. The process is difficult, emotionally draining, and complex for parents. An understanding of programmatic variables can be utilized to evaluate programs and programmatic outcomes.

SUMMARY

This chapter described the "anatomy" of a program in terms of its philosophical and programmatic components. The philosophical approach of any program represents the foundation of educational services and goals. The philosophy connects all of the teachers, specialists, and parents together with programming activities. The philosophy of a program is its reason for generating specific goals and performing selected activities. The philosophy of a program describes why certain types of disabled children require specific teachers, goals, and activities.

Language-disordered preschool children need to be recognized with a language-based philosophical approach in education. They also need a language pathologist in the classroom and a language-based learning curriculum that will facilitate language learning skills. The significant people in their lives must be offered parent-education programs. The success of any program must be directly related to children's development. The child must be the measure of educational success; programs must be modified based on the assessment of the child. The curriculum, the goals, the activities, everything in a school needs to tie into an underlying philosophy and ultimately be measured by changes in the child.

A FEW WORDS FROM TOYA DAVIS

I would like to share with you my thoughts and feelings about one of the issues raised in this chapter. I am the parent of two children, both of whom had developmental disabilities of one kind or another. As you know, my son Jonathan had a severe language and communication disorder. When I first recognized that Jonathan had serious learning problems I had no idea what that actually meant. One issue in this chapter is learning to understand the life-cycle process in terms of a special-needs child.

It was hard to imagine at age three when Jonathan was a preschooler what would be ahead or what he would be like when he was ten or fifteen or twenty. I had all kinds of hopes and dreams and expectations for him. All of these were shaken by my realization that he had a language disorder. What would this mean in the future? Would it mean that he would never be in a regular class? Would it mean that he would never have friends? Would it mean that he would never get married? Who would assure me of what would lie ahead in the future?

My husband, Arthur, and I had to learn to talk to each other about Jonathan. We had to learn to share our thoughts, our feelings, and our fears about this child that we love so much. Facing the future means accepting Jonathan in the present. There were many problems and issues that came up over the past eight years. In learning to understand Jonathan I was able to explain things to him so that he would understand and not be frightened and confused. I have always said that Jonathan taught me a great deal about being a mother and a person. Jonathan was not just a child with a language disorder; he was a child who taught me a great deal about myself.

REFERENCES

Alvin, J. (1975). *Music therapy.* London: John Clare Books.

Alvin, J. (1976). *Music for the handicapped child.* New York: Oxford University Press.

The American Association for Music Therapy, P.O. Box 80012, Valley Forge, PA 19484

The American Dance Therapy Association, 2000 Century Plaza, Suite 108, Columbia, MD 21044

The American Occupational Therapy Association, P.O. Box 1725, Rockville, MD 20849-1725

The American Psychological Association, 750 First St., N.E., Washington, DC 20002-4242

The American Speech Language Hearing Association, 10801 Rockville Pike, Rockville, MD 20852

Anderson, J. (1986). Sensory intervention with the preterm infant in the neonatal intensive care unit. *American Journal of Occupational Therapy, 40*(1), 19–26.

Bailey, D. B., Simeonsson, R. J., Yoder, D., & Huntington, G. S. (1990). Preparing professionals to serve infants and toddlers with handicaps and their families: An integrative analysis across eight disciplines. *Exceptional Children, 57*, 26–35.

Baker, B. L. (1984). Intervention with families with young, severely handicapped children. In J. Blacher (Ed.), *Severely handicapped young children and their families: Research in review.* Orlando, FL: Academic Press, Inc.

Boxhill, E. (1985). *Music therapy for the developmentally disabled.* Rockville, MD: Aspen Systems.

Bruscia, K. (1989). *Defining music therapy.* Spring City, PA: Spring House Books.

Deal, A. G., Dunst, C. J., & Trivette, C. M. (1989). A flexible and functional approach to developing individualized family support plans. *Infants and Young Children, 1*, 32–43.

Dunst, C. J., Johanson, C., Trivette, C. M., Hamby, D. (1991). Family-oriented early intervention policies and practices: family-centered or not? *Exceptional Child, 58*, 115–125.

Ekstein, R. (1983). *Children of Time and Space, of Action and Impulse.* New York: Jason Aronson, Inc.

Gillet, P. (1993). *Auditory processes revised.* Novato, CA: Academic Therapy Publications, Inc.

Giangreco, M., York, J., & Rainforth, B. (1989). Providing related services to learners with severe handicaps in educational settings: Pursuing the least restrictive option. *Pediatric Physical Therapy, 1,* 55–63.

Greenspan, S., & Pollock, G. (1989). *The Course of Life, Vol. II. Early Childhood.* Madison, CT: International Universities Press, Inc.

Hains, A. H., Rosenkoetter, S. E. , Fowler, S. A. (1991). Transition planning with families in early intervention. *Infants and Young Children, 3,* 38–47.

Hanft, B., & Humphry, R. (1989, April). Training occupational therapists in early intervention. *Infants and Young Children, 1,* 54–66.

Hopkins, H. (1988). An historical perspective on occupational therapy. In H. Hopkins & H. Smith (Eds.), *Willard & Spackman's occupational therapy.* Philadelphia: Lippincott.

Levy, F. J. (1992). *Dance movement therapy: A healing art.* Reston, VA: The American Alliance for Health, Physical Education, Recreation and Dance.

Lowell, E. L., & Stoner, M. (1960). *Play it by ear! Auditory training games.* Los Angeles: Wolfer Publishing Co.

Nordoff, P., & Robbins, C. (1971). *Therapy in music for handicapped children.* London: Gollancz.

Northcott, W. H. (1984). *Hearing Impaired Children, Birth to 3 years and their parents.* (Curriculum guide.) Washington, DC: The Alexander Graham Bell Association for the Deaf, Inc.

Ploof, D. L., & Feldman, H. M. (1992). Organizing early intervention services in a hospital setting: The Developmental Support Project as a parallel organization. *Infants and Young Children: An Interdisciplinary Journal of Special Care Practices, 5,* 28–39.

Reynolds, C. R., & Gutkin, T. B. (1990). *The handbook of school psychology*, 2nd ed. New York: John Wiley & Sons.

Salvia, J., & Ysseldyke, J. (1991). *Assessment,* 5th ed. Boston: Houghton Mifflin Co.

Sattler, J. M. (1988). *Assessment of children,* 3rd ed. San Diego: Jerome M. Sattler.

Stern, D. (1985). *The interpersonal world of the infant.* New York: Basic Books, Inc.

Tingey, C. (1989). *Implementing Early Intervention.* Baltimore: Paul H. Brookes Publishing Co.

Wilbarger, W. (1984). Planning an adequate "sensory diet"—Application of sensory processing theory during the first year of life. *Zero to Three, 5*(1), 7–12.

Williamson, G. (1988). Motor control as a resource for adaptive coping. *Zero to Three, 9,* 1–7.

Wright, J. S., Granger, R. D., & Sameroff, A. J. (1984). Parental acceptance and developmental handicap. In J. Blacher (Ed.), *Severely handicapped young children and their families.* Orlando, FL: Academic Press.

INDEX